WHOLE
& FREE
HEALTH

WHOLE & FREE HEALTH

YOUR GUIDE TO A HEALTHY
WEIGHT AND HAPPIER YOU
IN BODY, SOUL, AND SPIRIT

JENDAYI HARRIS

Emotional Fitness Trainer

ISBN: 978-0-9971867-9-6

Library of Congress Control Number:

Classification: LCC RC552.E18 | DDC 616.8526–dc22

Cover: Whole & Free Press
Interior: Wordzworth
Editors: Sarah Hayhurst & Bree J. Schuette

Printed in the United States of America.

Published by:
Whole & Free Press
P. O. Box 371391
Denver, CO 80237

DEDICATION

With Great Love To:

My Source, my All,
Words cannot express my love and gratitude.

To My Mothers:

Joann, Thank you for your incredible generosity, and for being
my one and only biological mom. I love you immensely.

Lorianne, Thank you for seeing the vision,
believing in me, and encouraging me without fail.

Debbie, Thank you for laboring with me
to get to the front line of my ministry.

My grandmothers, *Josephine* and *Ada,* I cherish you.

In Loving Memory and Honor:

My grandfather, *Ellis E. Harris, Senior,* Thank you
for filling the gap. You were my favorite eating buddy.

DISCLAIMER

Jendayi Harris, Whole & Free Press, Next Level Therapy, Llc.
Disclaimer for Whole & Free Health Book Contents.

This book, its content and any linked material are presented for informational purposes only and are not a substitute for medical advice, diagnosis, treatment, or prescribing. Nothing contained in or accessible from this book should be considered to be medical advice, diagnosis, treatment, or prescribing, or a promise of benefits, claim of cure, legal warranty, or guarantee of results to be achieved. Never disregard medical advice or delay in seeking it because of something you have read in this book. Neither Jendayi Harris, nor Whole & Free Press, nor Next Level Therapy Llc is a medical doctor or other licensed healthcare practitioner or provider. Consult with a licensed healthcare professional before altering or discontinuing any current medications, treatment or care, or starting any diet, exercise or supplementation program, or if you have or suspect you might have a health condition that requires medical attention. The United States Food and Drug Administration has not evaluated any statement, claim, or representation made in or accessible from this book or any linked material. The content of this book is not guaranteed to be correct, complete, or up-to-date. Whole & Free Health e-book especially may contain links to other resources on the Internet. These links are provided as citations and aids to help you identify and locate other Internet resources that may be of interest, and are not intended to state or imply that Jendayi Harris or Next Level Therapy, Llc or Whole and Free Press recommends, endorses, supports, sponsors, or is in any way affiliated or associated with any person or entity associated with the linked material, or is legally authorized to use any trade name, registered trademark, logo, legal or official seal, or copyrighted symbol that may be reflected in the linked material. If you would like to communicate with us, please email *info@wholeandfreepress.com*.

Note: All references to diabetes refer to type 2 diabetes, not type 1 diabetes.

Disclosure: Remember to consider all advice with a medical doctor. The author and any affiliation with this book are not held liable for health recommendations.

TABLE OF FREEDOM

Download Your Free
Call to Weight & Eating Freedom Action Plan
www.thechubbychurch.com

FREEDOM FRIES AND SUPER-SIZED LIES

—KRISTEN YANEY—

Freedom doesn't taste like French fries
Freedom doesn't taste like hot dogs or melted ice cream
That's congealed at the bottom of a soggy cardboard container
Because it got left out on your kitchen counter

Freedom, I promise you, Does not contain —
Hydrogenated oils, aspartame, nor sodium
sterol lactylate as a processing aid
Freedom doesn't taste like sadness
Freedom doesn't taste small
Freedom doesn't smell like those pretzels you get at the mall

So now that you know what Freedom is not
You probably realize that it can't be store bought
Not even at Whole Foods or Trader Joes
Though there's plenty of Brands that would sell you those

Freedom is not a commodity to be sold
Freedom is something you already own
Freedom is the birthright of your soul
Freedom is the hunger you seek, for it will satiate your every need
Freedom does just that — it breaks free!

Freedom tastes like velvety layers of cream
Sweet enough to coat the bitterness of good coffee
Sweeping over your tongue
Freedom tastes like drinking in Victory when the Battle is Won

Freedom tastes like a breath of fresh air on a cool Autumn day
While you lay back resting on a bale of sweet hay
Freedom tastes like Summer days stretched out at the park
Playing Frisbee with your friends until it gets dark

It tastes like you're running, wild and free
It feels like you're finally swimming downstream
It feels like you're patient, and done playing small
It feels like your heart finally knocked down the walls
It feels like your soul just cannot be contained
To be honest it feels… well, it feels kind of strange

It feels like you've finally conquered the lies
It feels like you've stood up and reclaimed your life
It feels like a fantastical, glorious feat
It feels like your soul wants to Dance to the Beat!
Freedom is shouting out, "Yes God, Yes God!"
Freedom feels like the rest of the time here on Earth
Is just getting started; a total rebirth!

What once was old, has been made new again
Freedom tastes like you're ready to Ascend

Follow Kristen Yaney on Medium
https://deeplyfunny.medium.com/
freedom-fries-and-super-sized-lies-1b633c1c658b

INTRODUCTION

Are you, too, a health enthusiast who struggles with weight and eating? Have you tried diet books, pills, or personal trainers only to gain more weight? Do you struggle with emotional eating, bingeing, or sugar addiction? Are you distressed about your eating habits leading you to chronic diseases such as pre-diabetes, heart disease, or cancer?

We're going over the mountain of what I call weight and eating bondage to weight and eating freedom. Bondage is slavery. For us it's being held captive by donuts, diets, or the number on the scale.

In **Whole & Free Health**, I'll walk you through freedom strategies for permanent weight release, more energy, and increased overall wellbeing with your eating plan of choice. If we drop weight with the latest diet fad, the bondage will still be alive on the inside, and we'll be challenged again. That's why 90 to 95 percent of people who lose weight regain it and then some.1

Here we'll make a conscious decision to get free from weight and eating bondage for good—for life. In Chapters 1-4 I'll set the stage for you to make sure you're in the right place to understand the importance of body, soul, and spirit to break free.

Then in Chapter 5 we'll complete **The Call to Weight & Eating Freedom Action Plan** to keep us motivated and inspired for taking corrective action toward our best health.

Instead of diets which are a distraction to the lifestyle changes that need to be made, in the Body section, Chapters 6-13, we'll work to **Master Body Care** with the Body H.A.B.I.T.S. which are foundational to great health and a healthy body weight such as nutrient loading, cleansing, and hormonal balancing. Mastering your body care will naturally lead you to reduce weight, prioritize yourself, and be happier when you look in the mirror.

We'll also gain an understanding of our soul's psychology in weight and eating bondage. These insights will help us find the hidden reasons we sabotage progress, eat like there's no food supply, and beat ourselves up over the damage.

In the Soul section, Chapters 14-19, you'll learn the psychological reasons that you use food to meet unmet needs and allow your inner glutton to sabotage you in **Grubbology**. Then we'll do deep reflection on why we self-protect with weight in **Chubbology**. I'm excited to teach you strategies for healing emotional eating episodes so you just can't binge anymore if you wanted to with an **Emotional Fitness Workout**. And gain insights to **Jump Off the Body Shame Train in Looksology**.

We'll wrap up with **Keys to Whole & Free Health**.

I know what it's like to feel absolutely hopeless that my weight would ever change, that my mind would be forever held hostage by its obsession with my next meal and wonder if I'd ever really like kale. I know what it's like to be a slave to food, a slave to cultural body image, a slave to the scale's report, and a slave to fear.

In my role as a therapist, I work with eating disordered clients who desperately needed the content to walk the healing path to weight and eating freedom, which I laid out in The Chubby Church Books 1 & 2.

The problem: all of my clients aren't Chubby Church members, and many carried some form of church hurt from their upbringing or were of other faiths and didn't resonate with a Christian audience.

So, I wrote Whole & Free Health to give the key insights that will ground you in essentials to weight, eating, food, and body image freedom.

However, spiritual health and inclusion is a major part of the transformation process. And I must disclose that I am in my core a lover of Jesus Christ and consider myself a non-denominational, spirit-led, non-judgmental, Christ follower. I honor your faith or lack thereof, but of course it's my heart for you to know the love of God. I also at times may get preachy and use Biblical references. My intention is not to offend you, but to give you tools that are powerful to promote your freedom.

The goal here is to include all of ourselves – body, soul, and spirit – to heal and grow through weight and eating issues.

Buddhists, Jews, and others have found the insight useful and supportive to their goals. Whatever your faith, I highly recommend you incorporate your views of God, Spirit, and spirituality to utilize the practical insights for a healthier, Whole & Free version of yourself.

When I mention Book 2, I am referring to *The Chubby Church* **Book 2:** *An Order to Win the 7 Battles of the Weight & Eating War for Good! As it's a necessary follow up to fully be free If you've been up and down in weight all of your life.*

As you turn the pages of this book, know that I deeply care and resonate with the struggle with food, body image, weight gain, dieting, and binge eating.

I cried on my knees several times in gratitude and awe that I was F-R-E-E from mental and emotional anguish, even though I don't have a fitness model body. In fact, I have strategically optimized cushioning, compliments of my African American heritage.

Are you willing to do what it takes to overcome your weight and eating battle for good? Will you commit to your freedom? Just go ahead and say, "Yes!"

Jendayi Harris

Soul Freedom Author & Speaker
Lover of God
Licenced Professional Counselor in Colorado
National Board Certified Counselor
Board-Certified Holistic Health Coach
Friend of the People

Email: *info@wholeandfreepress.com*
www.jendayiharris.com | www.nextleveltherapyllc.com
www.thechubbychurch.com | www.wholeandfreeu.com

· CHAPTER 1 ·

IS THIS FOR ME? QUIZ

Next time you see someone with a nice body who looks like he or she just walked out of the Garden of Eden, think to yourself, I look like that under here.

For years, I struggled with what I call bondage to weight and eating without thinking about the bigger picture. I needed more insight than diet advice telling me to eat cottage cheese and work out.

I had no idea I had a god named McNuggets, accompanied by worship practices that included fries and hot mustard sauce. I was a slave to feel good food and the health consequences thereof.

I emotionally ate and ate and ate.

I battled diet after diet, ate fast food three times a day, and lost and gained weight several times. How frustrating to win in other areas of life but feel like a loser in the weight and eating battle, over and over again.

Then one day, in much agony over weight and eating struggles after losing less than expected on a thirty day juice fast, I parked my car and laid my head on the steering wheel.

This time you'll need to do things My way.

Tears streamed down my cheeks as Spirit whispered. My diet shenanigans needed to retire. I faced a problem my education, knowledge of health, and spiritual study alone couldn't solve.

You'll get permanent instead of temporary.

I listened to that still, small voice. Permanent sounded much better than the dramatic up and down weight woes I experienced for the past decade.

Freedom, Yes, Freedom

Much of my heart and mental energy was spent trying to figure out what I wanted to eat or the weight I needed to lose. In 2004, I was fifty pounds overweight from eating fast food three times a day, yet I wondered why I had symptoms of weight gain, disgusting greenish black fungal issues on my skin, irritable bowel syndrome, moodiness, depression, fatigue, bad acne, psoriasis, and asthma.

But worst of all, a tormented mind harassed me like a pre-teen who wants a cell phone. It drove me to think I needed to lose weight, even at times when I didn't. At that time, my mind demanded fatty, sugary, doughy foods and took my focus from other plans for my life.

Spirit led me to holistic nutrition, allowed me to lose over fifty pounds, and delivered me from traditional fast food.

A miracle of the modern age.

Yet, along the way, I somehow regained the weight because the problem wasn't just the food. In fact, I'll share with you in Chapter 3 how I regained the pounds by eating organic cookies and snacks.

Three times, I've lost and gained significant poundage. So, I'm not sure if I'm an expert on weight gain or weight loss at this point, but either way, I'm happy to help.

My body reflected my soul. And I now know it was my soul weight that really needed to get lost. Soul weight is our brokenness, grief, financial anxiety, anger, and insecurity.

Yes, our inner transformation allows for body revelation.

I found the path to freedom from the bondage of weight and eating. As I learned to seek physical, emotional, mental, and spiritual

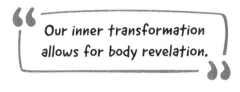

> Our inner transformation allows for body revelation.

health, I was able to not only release weight, but become Whole & Free.

Are You Ready to be Whole & Free?

Do you struggle with weight and eating? Have you tried diet books, pills, or personal trainers only to gain more weight? Do you struggle with emotional eating, overeating, or sugar addiction? Are you wondering why God just won't help you with your weight even after you've prayed a hundred times?

I call this struggle: weight and eating bondage. It's a complex issue that I've simplified to help you move out of bondage to Whole & Free Health.

Let's make sure you're in the right place.

WEIGHT & EATING BONDAGE QUIZ

Mark each statement below that resonates with you:

1. I feel out of control with certain foods, ingredients, and/or drinks. ☐

2. I often overeat and stuff myself with food. ☐

3. I undereat, skip meals, and often neglect my nutritional needs. ☐

4. I have poor health. ☐

5. I've had surgery to help me lose weight. ☐

6. I don't like my body. ☐

7. I often criticize and obsess about certain body parts. ☐

8. I avoid looking at myself in mirrors. ☐

9. I always want to lose weight, but I don't get any lasting results even when I try. ☐

10. I often work out but then eat poorly after my workout. ☐

11. I exercise primarily to lose weight. ☐

12. I fast with the main motive of losing weight gained from poor eating. ☐

13. I often obsess over my health and weight condition. ☐

14. I fear getting a disease. ☐

15. I frequently crave sugary, salty, fatty, or floury foods. ☐

16. I eat quickly—a full plate is gone in less than five to ten minutes. ☐

17. I am considered overweight or obese. ☐

18. I've been diagnosed with an eating disorder. ☐

19. I've gained and lost weight over twenty pounds more than once in my life. ☐

20. I feel my weight blocks me from living my best life. ☐

Total Score:

**Any statement marked is a sign
you're reading the right book.**

_____

This book is for the chronic dieter, the fast food junkie, and the binger. The man or woman threatened with heart disease or diabetes because of eating habits. It's for the woman who got gastric bypass years ago only to gain it all back and then some. The guy obsessed with his leg muscles. And for the person scared they'll get cancer again if they don't change their eating habits.

And you don't have to be chubby to read this book. Plenty of skinny fat people are popping lots of pills and chomping on bottomless bags of chips. Many are normal weight but in weight and eating bondage.

Whatever your story, I'm glad you want to do something about it.

There's no condemnation here, and this isn't about shaming you because of the candy bar you ate yesterday. It's about you emotionally, mentally, and spiritually maturing into a person who can stand fully in love for your true self. It's about freedom from that little god in your belly who demands your attention and takes you away from being emotionally and physically available to what matters.

Again, inner transformation brings body revelation.

So, the next time you see someone with a nice body who looks like they just walked out of the Garden of Eden, think to yourself, *I look like that under here*, because the physical body you want is already there, waiting to be revealed.

Thankfully, we don't need false weapons of liposuction, diet potions, or a will power ax to win the battle. What we need are solid strategies, mindsets, skills, and principles for health. No matter what your size or how long you've struggled with weight and eating, victory is yours!

Please don't just read this book: read it through quickly, then read Book 2, and study them both. You'll have the principles to become the best version of yourself on the inside, which in turn will manifest on the outside.

What's Been Missing?

Clearly, why you haven't succeeded before isn't because God doesn't love you or want you to succeed. It's not because you're born to be fat or inherit disease.

The world misleads us on this topic of weight and eating just like with most other things. The world says being a size two is successful and worthy of love. Not true! You're loved no matter your shape and size.

This isn't about being a size two or having a thirty four inch waist. It doesn't mean you have to start a crash diet today or give up cake forever. It's not my mission to be the food police. And, for the record, it's not the size of a person that determines their freedom. Some of us are naturally bigger than others and naturally carry more weight.

It's also not all about being overweight or obese. Plenty of folks are a normal weight but are still not paying adequate attention to proper nutrition and take diet induced blood pressure, cholesterol, or diabetes medications. No matter what your state of health or shape, you're so much more than your body shape and size!

I believe that freedom is being emotionally, spiritually, physically, and mentally healthy and engaged with life. See, the world says, "Diet, diet, and diet some more," yet dieting gets you big, bigger, and the biggest you've ever been in your life!

Because diets don't look at the deeper root cause but only symptoms. Which, as a result, leads you on the search for another diet. This is soul extortion from the father of lies. It's demoralizing to go on and off diets, to win and lose the weight battle over and over again.

The world is deceptive, but the biggest deception is who you really are as a child of God. The real you isn't chubby, nor is the real you subject to torment in thinking you're not healthy enough, good looking enough, or good enough.

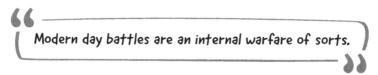

Modern day battles are an internal warfare of sorts.

Weight and eating struggles don't mean that you're defective or a piglet. Weight and eating freedom is a measurement tool of how much you're growing in as your authentic, healthy self.

You're blessed because you will see your growth and transformation from the inside to the outside. And, you're not alone. We've all got something to overcome, right?

Battles were gruesome back in the day when natives had to defeat real giants with arrows. Modern day battles are an internal warfare of sorts. We battle enemies of our own soul's mind, will, and emotions as well as spirit and body.

Once you're in agreement with unhealthy living, hating your body, abusing your body with food, hanging out on the hamster wheel of dieting, or absolute inertia from making a change out of obesity, there's nothing more for the lies in your mind to do. You've lost, and they've won because the lies are internalized. In other words, you believe what you repeat in your head several times a day, even if it's a lie.

No more will you be subject to these destructive lies.

As we move through the material, you'll become equipped with knowledge, wisdom and understanding, practical application, and real strategies to win for life.

What to Expect

This isn't a diet book. Diet books only work for a limited time. I'm interested in your complete freedom and wellness for life. Unlike weight loss books that give specific diet guidelines to follow or make you feel like it just takes your willpower to *shape up , you bad, bad dieter, you*, this book does neither. This book offers no shame and certainly no unrealistic rice cake diet or any diet at all for that matter.

I have no stones to throw.

The promise in this book is weight and eating freedom. This is an "I want to take my life and health out of lies and into the truth and appreciate my body and be my true self." type of book. I want you to be free at any weight. I outline the exact thinking, skills, and understanding to get you there, but take it one bite at a time.

I hope you get that it isn't about looking great in swim trunks or a bikini, but about being healthy for the highest good for your life.

You may cry with real thanksgiving, as my clients have, that you have been set free. I cried on my knees several times in gratitude and awe that I was F-R-E-E, even though I don't have a fitness model body. In fact, I have strategically optimized cushioning, compliments of my African American heritage.

Let's get to it.

REFLECT & SHARE

1. What did the weight and eating bondage quiz reveal to you?

_____

_____

_____

_____

2. Why do you care about your weight and eating freedom?

_____

_____

_____

_____

CHAPTER 2

GAINING WHOLE & FREE HEALTH

We know deep down we're digging
our graves faster with a knife and fork.

Everyone knows by now that certain food choices will lead you to heaven faster. So, why are we choosing them? Why is it so difficult to control?

I believe it's because America is on a highway to obesity and disease. The Centers for Disease Control and Prevention report that one half of the American population will be obese by 2030.[1] In 1980, 15 percent of American adults were obese, and in 2016 that number was 38.9 percent.[2,3] I wish stocks doubled like that—but people, not so thrilling. It's already the case that more than a third of us are overweight and a third are obese. Researchers estimate the growing obesity figures will result in up to an additional $66 billion dollars in health care expenditures, 7.8 million new cases of diabetes, 6.8 million new cases of stroke and heart disease, and more than 500,000 new cancer diagnoses per year.[4]

Bondage is expensive.

Yet we know that you don't have to be obese to be in bondage to poor food choices, binge eat, or obsess about weight.

The Standard American Diet (notice its acronym S.A.D.) is an eating disorder in and of itself. Currently, most Americans eat less than

12 percent fruits and vegetables and over 80 percent processed or highly processed foods.[5, 6] This leaves many in a state of slavery to food tempta-

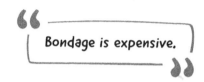

Bondage is expensive.

tion, be inactive, overeat, or drive the body to be thin. And it's far from nature's instructions to eat mostly plants for food and meat, birds, and fish if we desired to.

Our lack of quality macronutrients (proteins, complex carbohydrates, and fat), combined with a severe micronutrient malnourishment (vitamins and minerals), are contributing to extensive health prayer requests and an abundance of medication, robbing Americans of the energy needed for quality of life.

The alluring practices of the food and drug industry are pushed by the media to tempt you. Then the media has the nerve to tell you that you're fat and to get on the latest diet pill. Not only that, but in the Body section, I'll explain the habits we need for better health. And it's not move more and eat less that solves our weight issues. That's the industries' way of putting their lack of responsibility on us.

With a focus on health, not weight, we can correct our eating from human engineered foods to nature created foods to take back our health in body, soul, and spirit.

Spiritual knowledge is no match for the wounds of the soul nor is health knowledge or any other knowledge about what we *should* do.

Health knowledge is no match for the wounds of the soul.

Look at your local doctors or nurses: they know health, don't they? Yet, we can see they look just like the statistics, too.

The soul matters.

It needs healing as our mind, will, and emotions affect our choices—for good or for evil—in spite of what we know. And certainly, in spite of what we don't know.

Can you agree that we may know what to do for our health—eat vegetables, drink water, and exercise, but we don't do it? This is why previous weight loss attempts have been limited. Too many address weight and eating from a one or two dimensional physical perspective, such as, "How many calories should I eat?" or, "How long should I do cardio to lose weight?"

When we struggle with weight and eating, it's much more than the physical. A traditional diet book can help in a limited way because it only addresses a part of the problem. The body, soul, and spirit operate together. We can't look at only the body and attempt to force it into better health and weight without looking at the motivations driving the soul.

> "
> **The body, soul, and spirit operate together.**
> "

Body manipulation is all those attempts you've made in the past to lose weight by working out and eating only lettuce for breakfast.

Manipulation is unsustainable.

We need to address psychological and spiritual aspects of weight and eating with fresh perspectives on the physical, too.

You create your life and body with the choices you make. And sadly, like I said, it's extremely difficult to make sound choices when your food supply is engineered to get you addicted to it.

Help Me to See What I Don't Want to See

To come into reality and talk about this is the first step to being free. We must come out of denial. We can pretend all we want that our eating habits don't matter, our body isn't important, or our weight doesn't reflect our soul, but we know deep down that we're digging our graves faster with a knife and fork.

Denial is the psychological phenomenon of being unable to see or admit the truth staring you in the face. Webster's dictionary calls it an unconscious, defense mechanism characterized by refusal to acknowledge painful realities, thoughts, or feelings.[7]

People who walk in denial have an invisible shield of protection from truth and reality. They continually live in a state of fantasy and

> **Poor self-care now will demand time from our loved ones and medical care later.**

victimization caused by avoiding making real changes. They aren't truly alive or engaged with life. They're like a zombie on *The Walking Dead*—blind that eating habits, food choices, and body criticisms create an unhealthy reality.

And when in denial, we live in a vacuum and can't see that our actions and inactions affect others in big and small ways. There's always an elephant in the room. We can't continue to be selfish by mismanaging our health. And poor self-care now will demand time from our loved ones and medical care later.

Would you agree, it's difficult to live your best life when you're caught up in chronic health issues stemming from weight and eating obsession?

Seriously, Spanx™ can only do so much. Eventually, we need to decide to deal with the way we use food to cope with life, hide in our emotions, and protect ourselves with that extra layer of chub.

It's time to let go of denial—the denial of thinking that another diet is the answer or that it's God's fault you're in the chubby suit you've created. It's time to accept that poor food choices create problems for you, your family, your purpose, and your health destiny. The fact of the matter is only you can decide to do something about it.

To break out of denial one of my favorite bold prayers is, "help me to see what I don't want to see."

This prayer will help you grow like a wildflower. Often, we shut down from addressing reality. Be bold, look in the mirror and accept the good, the bad, and the ugly. To walk in victory of Whole & Free Health.

REFLECT & SHARE

1. How have you been in denial about your weight and eating bondage?

_____

_____

_____

_____

_____

_____

_____

_____

_____

_____

CHAPTER 3

WELCOME TO BURGER KING
MY STORY

I realized I had a problem when
I was a slave to the Burger King.

Before we dig into things, I'll share the details of my story with you for three reasons. First, when we connect to our stories, we lay a stronger foundation for lasting change. Second, my story is used throughout this book to help you apply the principles. And third, it's easier to connect more dots in your own story when you hear and can relate to someone else's story. So, here it goes.

For over three months in 2003, I couldn't break free from Burger King's chocolate-chip cookies, which really put a dent in my perpetual diet. I was trapped in a vicious cycle. It happened like this; on the drive to work at my new job as a financial advisor, I stopped at Burger King and got a cookie or two at 8 a.m. Don't tell my kid nephew this, but yes, I ate cookies for breakfast. On the way home from work, I'd get another one at around 8 p.m. Some days, I went for a lunchtime cookie fix, too.

Perhaps a job on *Sesame Street* would have been better suited because I was the biggest cookie monster on the block.

Besides the ooey, gooey, chocolatey taste bud party and the intoxicating aroma, I had no consciousness of why I ate the cookies. *Sure, I thought, I deserve these, I'm stressed.* But no real answers came to mind—only excuses. Did I even want an answer? Not really. A part of me liked eating those cookies, a rather large part. I enjoyed my daily worship routine as I pulled up to the drive through window.

"Welcome to Burger King. Can I take your order?," said the worker.

At 230 calories a pop and with a desire to lose weight, I wanted to stop this cycle but found myself answering that question every single day. Out of the burger kingdom temptation called. I wanted to serve the King of Kings, not the Burger King. I needed deliverance from a cookie! Finally, a new commute from an office move got this cookie demon off my back. But my cookie freedom only lasted a little while.

Victory at Last ... So I Thought

My cookie stops turned into fast food meals three times a day, which fast tracked me to a two week sick leave from work for bronchitis, amongst a host of other strange things happening to my body. I did what any twenty something year old would do: I went home to mama who lived about ninety minutes away for a reprieve.

It was there that a life changing moment came in the restroom. I saw a book in my peripheral vision entitled *Natural Cures They Don't Want You to Know About. Who is they?* I certainly wanted to know. I coughed uncontrollably as I leaned over to pick it up. Intrigued, I thumbed through it. As I skimmed the pages that talked about nutrition, I thought, *Could I be sick because of my diet?*

Barely able to breathe, I hobbled down the hall to my bedroom with my eyes fixed on the book. The book's wisdom invited me into a sense of God's presence.

I sat on the bed, and for a moment I enjoyed the sunlight through the window as the warmth embraced my face. I didn't recall the last time I had sat in the sun. I couldn't remember the last time I read a book.

Where have I been? Eighty hours of work a week was likely the culprit. *Oh yeah,* I realized as though a light bulb glowed over my head, *I'm sick because I'm a workaholic and maybe my diet.* At that time to think I was a food addict was incomprehensible despite the obvious signs. Denial is a doozie.

As I read, I reflected on my health. My air supply randomly cut off, it took me at least an hour to get out of bed in the morning, and I wheezed in between every other word. Not feeling too healthy. Not to mention the extra poundage I carried around. I longed for my energetic lean runner's body from college weight loss efforts.

I was beyond out of control.

The lines struck me as I read: "But once the food is processed and put in a box or a can, you're going to have to eat 100 times more to get the same nutritional value; nutrition is virtually wiped out. So, in addition to having the poisons put in your system from the chemicals not even listed on the label, the food you are getting has almost no nutritional value."[1]

Unbelievable, I thought. I hadn't known anything about nutrition. *Could this be true?* It was about dinner time. On a mission of truth … or camouflaged addiction, I drove to my favorite fast food establishment. *Is fast food empty food with no nutritional value?* I should know. I ate it three times per day for weeks on end.

"I'll take the nuggets and fries meal with sweet and sour sauce, please." With an ear to ear grin, I picked up my experimental meal. As a fast food junkie, I relaxed into my daily worship practice and ate on the way back to mom's house. And twenty-three minutes later, I was hungry again. My brain seemed to want more nuggets. My stomach felt empty. But my belly could've been mistaken for a round pool float.

It was December 28, 2004. The sacred date of my last traditional fast food meal.

I read. All night. Amazed.

But, when I rose the next day, panic set in. *What in the world was I going to eat?!* I had to go to the dreaded grocery store.

Oh, God. I thought, as I stared at the bright tomatoes, carrots, and green vegetables I didn't know existed. Bewildered, red nosed, and hacking, I thought, *I could live off chicken soup this week. But what would I eat next week? Grapefruits.* I was clueless as my diet was 100 percent processed foods with a dismal array of cooking skills.

My journey over the next few months astounded me and my colleagues. I went from fast food junkie to whole-clean-slow foods and lost fifty pounds.

My strange symptoms disappeared and were replaced by a vibrant glow so bright my colleagues and their spouses signed up to learn about health from me. Overnight I had a health coaching business. It felt amazing to support people in such a meaningful way. I read incessantly about health, whole foods, and nutrition. A natural passion awakened.

I thought I'd never have a weight problem again.

Never say never.

The Return of the Cookie Demon

My diet had transformed to eat healthier, organic, whole foods until a new relationship. Turns out my *inner glutton* was in remission during my health revelation. The threat of falling in love when I met my fiancé sparked deep insecurities. Love felt worse than tight underwear on backwards in a work meeting—awful.

Naturally, I made regular trips to buy large, organic, chocolate-chip cookies from Whole Foods Market. Sounds healthier, doesn't it? Certainly, but no less fattening nor less insulin spiking.

When I became engaged, it got worse. My insecurities around closeness made me eat more. And I didn't hide it either. Before a long drive my mother made homemade cookies for my fiancé and me. There were forty freshly baked, chocolate-chip cookies for us to share. By the time we drove the two-and-a-half-hours to Maryland from New Jersey, the cookies were gone! Like Houdini. Not a crumb in sight. The cookie-to-person ratio was an embarrassing 35:5, for each one he ate, I ate seven.

After marriage, the obsession morphed into a full-on compulsion. I ate whole boxes of cookies, now from a local bakery. By this time I knew all about health, food, and weight loss. I taught whole foods nutrition classes and coached people. I lost fifty pounds, not once but twice!

First, I did it with exercise in college. *Aha!* I thought at the time, *I could just work out every day to slim down.* Only after the slim down, I went back to being too busy to exercise.

Second, I lost it with body detoxification and healthy clean eating. *Aha!* I thought, *I could heal my body through nutrition and cleansing.* After some time, the pounds boomeranged back. *Hmm, maybe there's more to this eating and exercise thing.* I admit, I'm not always the sharpest pencil in the box.

As the baked goods frenzy amplified, so did my waistline. I gobbled cookies and prayed for weight loss at the same time. I was at a standstill, unable to solve the problem of weight and eating in my life.

I worked a twelve-step process. I'd go to the store, get cookies, eat cookies, feel bad, feel bloated, feel unhealthy, feel sad, feel demoralized, feel ashamed, feel lonely, and then had the audacity to go get and eat more cookies to feel better! I was entrapped. I'd eaten enough chocolate-chip cookies to last not only my lifetime but that of four generations after me, too.

Things didn't change until I wanted freedom from soul bondage *more* than I wanted the weight to fall off, and *more* than I wanted the object of my false comfort (cookies).

> **Things didn't change until I wanted freedom from soul bondage more than I wanted the weight to fall off, and more than I wanted the object of my false comfort.**

It was more than body weight I was wearing. I wore soul weight. I wore the weight of my past. I wore the weight of my sin. I ate my fears, anger, grief, lust, and insecurities.

I knew about health, I relied on the Lord, but no matter what I knew was right for me, my health knowledge was no match for the holes in my soul. I worked with God to find answers to heal my mindset, my fear of releasing weight for good, and the emotions underneath the compulsions.

> " Health knowledge was no match for the holes in my soul. "

These answers led me to permanent weight release, more energy, soul freedom, and a healthier, happier body and mind. The results of this weight and eating freedom only make the evidence of weight and eating bondage more obvious.

What Weight & Eating Freedom Is Like

Whether your cookie shows up as ice cream, potato chips, tortilla chips, chocolate, soda, coffee, cake, bread, pizza, or cookies, like me, freedom can begin.

The benefits of weight and eating freedom keep giving. It's a blessing to eat a piece of cake and not the whole cake. And when I do overeat, I provide myself compassion instead of berating myself, which used to lead me to eat more. I can now enjoy my body as weight fluctuates with hormones or age.

What a joy it is to fit comfortably into an airline seat or easily bend down to pick something up. How nice it is to see my feet when I look down or play airplane with a child with ease. I appreciate the freedom of not judging myself when I want to eat real food.

I fully appreciate who I am and know that I am more than how much I weigh. I know God loves me as I am. I am free to be me, and I am so much better in Him.

This soul freedom allows me to be honest with myself, as well as others, about what I think, how I feel, and what I need. I value myself just as much as anyone else. I'm no longer a doormat or a bulldozer. I matter. I believe I can handle life because God will sustain, help, and protect me at all times. This is true freedom. This is security. This is soul safety. Life uses weight and eating struggles to free us not only in body, but in soul and spirit.

Nothing tastes better than the whole and free you.

I wanted you to get a taste of what my freedom is like because it's all available for you, too. Imagine your freedom, and you'll see nothing tastes better than the whole and free you.

When Did This Start?

One of the best things my mother did for me was encourage me to get baptized at six years old. I remember talks with the Lord as a child throughout my tumultuous home life. There were moments I could touch His presence, although I didn't know how to use my faith to withstand the turmoil in my heart or home.

One night, my dad came home in a substance-induced rage. In a fit, he aggressively destroyed dishes, furniture, and whatever was in his path downstairs, while we slept upstairs. Scared, my mom snuck out their bedroom window onto the carport to get help.

Determined to end her struggle with domestic abuse with her troubled young husband once and for all, my mother rallied a few college kids to help her get us out. In the wee hours of the morning, we — my two brothers, and I — escaped through a broken window on the second floor through their master bedroom. We arrived at her parent's house a short drive away.

She was clear they'd be divorced as soon as possible. And they were.

My sensitive, six-year-old heart was overwhelmed with uncertainty. My earliest memories were filled with fear and anxiety in this chaotic place I called home. I witnessed my mother being disrespected, yelled at, or outright physically abused.

My dad was a good man. He was positive, inspiring, and encouraging.

But he was also tormented by adultery, alcohol, and a gripping cocaine addiction that brought out a violent side.

My parents' unresolved past hindered us all. Their explosive relationship caused consuming angst for me.

We left everything behind and lived with my grandparents. One night, my grandmother served sauerkraut and hot dogs for dinner. I hadn't experienced sauerkraut before, what a taste explosion! I stuffed it into my little mouth as fast as I could.

Three servings later, I didn't feel so good. And upchucked it all. Right there. At the table. It was gross, but my brain had found a way for me to cope with my emotional sensitivity. I had a solution for the depth of emotional pain I experienced in my chaotic young life: stuff the pain down with food! This was the beginning of a lifelong struggle with my new bestie: food.

We later moved to another suburb of New Jersey, across the street from a shopping center. Whenever I got money, I headed to the drug store to get a candy bar. Funny enough, the candy bar was my drug.

Bring on the paper route, because when I had some real money, you know ten bucks, I'd get mozzarella sticks from the local Friday's restaurant. Due to my habit of running to food since I was six years old, I didn't develop the tools to actually deal with my emotions.

Humans of all ages are meant to be seen, heard, and loved. If not, we usually deal with our need in unhealthy ways.

To make matters worse, six years later when I was twelve years old, we received headline news that struck like a tsunami.

The Root of the Cookie Craving

My two brothers and I sat at the kitchen table as we wondered, why did Aunt Lori sound so insistent for mom to call her back?

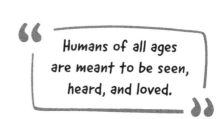

> Humans of all ages are meant to be seen, heard, and loved.

My older brother took my Aunt's call after my mom left in a frenzy to calm down that October day in our Marlton, New Jersey townhouse.

We were grateful our mom did come back. At times, with a stressed-out single mom, you just never knew.

She called Aunt Lori back.

"What is it?" my mom asked my dad's sister on the other line. Seconds later, she dropped the white corded phone and hunched over in shock.

A loud wail followed, "Aaagh!" and a dam of tears broke. Her mouth grasped for air between deep sobs. Time froze as tears kindled in all of us. My stomach queasy.

My father was found dead behind the back of a Camden, New Jersey, liquor store at the ripe age of thirty-four years old. He was murdered—shot right in the face. A black cloud descended as a gang of emotional hoodlums beat down my heart.

My wounds were already raw, yet a knife seemed to cut them deeper. The bleeding didn't stop. It was the worst day of my life.

Still is.

As the cloudy months followed, I baked. My chocolate-chip cookie cakes soothed my wounds. Distracted from grief, I baked cookie cakes for everyone.

I loved my daddy. But now, my beloved daddy was gone. I'd run, jump, and hug him every time I saw him as he greeted us in the driveway with his huge smile. I'd let out girlish giggles as he'd catch me and hold me close, even when I was big.

These special daddy-daughter moments happened every time we visited the six years between the scary night we left and the worst day of my life. I ate cookies for that hug. I chewed for that sense of safety.

Every sweet memory of the first man I ever loved was drowned with morsels of America's old-time favorite. I lost my daddy, but food was faithful. I never worried about it dying or rejecting me. Food was reliable. It didn't neglect me. It was there.

Over twenty years of my life were dedicated to solving my soul holes through eating and obsessing over food and weight. I plugged these holes with food so I could stay in denial about my pain. I attempted to diet it away countless times, but truth is persistent.

Weight gain was my absent father's protection. Overeating was my working, single mother's nurturance and comfort when I was home alone or fighting with my brothers for being knuckleheads over Nintendo. At first, my eating issues were a sound strategy, but by my teenage years, weight gain and hormones turned my obsession into torment.

The conflicting desires to eat whatever I wanted and look good hijacked my mind. My overeating left me unsatisfied, unfulfilled, and unhappy because self-harm always comes with a side portion of weight gain, shame, guilt, anxiety, and body dissatisfaction.

When my parents divorced, I desperately needed a loving hug, but it was food that would snuggle me. My eating measured the level of emotional pain I felt on the inside. My weight gain reflected the depth of insecurity and deep pain in my soul.

My addiction to the food obsession was an attempt to control and manipulate my out of control identity crisis, like a child seeking love and protection from a hamburger mistaken as mom and dad.

As I gained momentum, I wanted to live and be better, healed, whole, grounded, and disciplined. Faith helped me believe it was possible, even though I wasn't really sure it was possible.

My automatic emotional reaction to life was food. When life was difficult or joyous or boring, I found my comfort through food. What's your story?

Why We Use Food

Self-sabotaging habits with food help us to cope with life. We use food to manage strong feelings we've not had the tools to manage,

> " Food obsession was an attempt to control and manipulate my out of control identity crisis. "

such as loneliness, disappointment, anger, stress, ambiguity, and neglect.

Tough feelings can drive a person with eating issues right up to the drive through window. Our eating issues are a strategy that our psychology uses to help our soul's emotions. It starts having negative effects in our lives and in our relationships because it's a false form of love.

When we're dysfunctional with food, we're trying to gain love. The biochemical power of the brain and body that's tied to our emotions is strong.

We use food to self-medicate as an anodyne. We use it to stuff down, avoid, hide, numb, celebrate, and comfort.

> Dieting is a distraction that creates an illusion of change.

Where's My Miracle?

If you want to be a whole and free, authentic person, you must take back your power to respond and own your full self. To own our emotions, mindset, health, and eating habits is tough.

It's easier to be a victim of the cookies than to say no to them. It's easier to blame than it is to own our part. It's more comfortable to stay stuck than it is to grow up. I dieted and never actually made changes. I was interested in a healthy, slim body, but I wasn't committed to healthier habits—nor a healthier me.

Dieting is a distraction that creates an illusion of change, but when you look at the fruit of it, there's no supporting actions to create lasting change.

I, too, wanted to be zapped with deliverance from my weight and eating issue. Lord knows I cried out, "Deliver me, Lord!" believing it was possible to be instantaneously delivered by some weight loss miracle. *Where is a Benny Hinn Healing Crusade when you need one?*

My painful inner turmoil got the best of me. I felt frustrated, angry, confused, and hopeless around the whole matter. I felt trapped in a cement chair. At times I'd rather die than deal with my tormenting hell.

I felt stupid talking about it to anyone. And when I did, they didn't get it. "Eat right and exercise," they said. I felt like I was the only one with this craziness going on inside of me. It felt so shameful to wear extra poundage that I hardly wanted to go anywhere.

Our weight and eating issue is our measurement of our growth in receiving God's love for who He's made us to be. It's about your heart. It's not even about your weight or food, but we'll address both because both are a part of this multifarious condition.

Ultimately, food, health, and weight issues are a call to heal. It's our call into greater freedom. We're in bondage in body, soul, and spirit until we fully commit to wholeness and freedom.

REFLECT & SHARE

1. What was difficult for you growing up that you may still binge over?

    _____

    _____

2. When did your story with food struggles begin? When did you first notice it?

    _____

    _____

3. What new freedoms are you looking forward to as you conquer this battle?

    _____

    _____

• CHAPTER 4 •

DO YOU WANT FREEDOM WITH THAT?

Freedom in Body, Soul, and Spirit

When we don't like the fruit, we must look at the roots.

To understand the body, soul, and spirit's integration, I'd like you to imagine a glass.

The glass is your body, and in it is:

Red juice, your soul.

Water, your spirit.

Oil, the Holy Spirit.

What would happen if the glass broke? Right, we couldn't drink the liquid. What about if the glass cracked? The liquid would then leak out. In other words, an effect on one inevitably affects the other.

This research and insight comes from Watchman Nee's 600 page, three volume work *The Spiritual Man*.[1] A spiritual man as one whose soul is governed by the Spirit. Our goal is just that, our soul working through God's Spirit. We're the driver, but

> **We're the driver, but Spirit's our GPS.**

Spirit's our GPS. A spiritual man or woman follows Spirit's directions. The carnal man or woman doesn't, hasn't downloaded the app, or has a bad connection.

The process of transformation from a carnal to a spiritual sanctification. The word sanctify is to "set apart for particular use in a special purpose or work and to make holy or sacred."[2]

The heart of God is to sanctify us in body, soul, and spirit.

In previous attempts to take back your health, did you take your soul into account? The sanctification process? Your identity? Your beliefs? Or your past?

Or have you only approached it from a physical body perspective? Chances are you have overlooked the soul and spirit aspects in health.

We need to have a holistic approach to solve health dilemma. Let's review the functions of each.

Body – Instrument, Sensory, Sacred

Imagine the complexity of this miraculous collection of more than 37 trillion cells that are all multiplying, regenerating, and interacting twenty four hours a day.[3] Only Divine Intelligence could create this amazing vessel for us to dwell in.

God wants us to care for this precious gift He gave us to live in. How we take care of our body indicates how much we honor it and this irreplaceable gift. And for the record, this doesn't necessarily mean no flab, wrinkles, or on the flip-side looking like Hercules. And according to body mass index calculations, Hercules is obese!

I'm saying, the most high-end Tesla can't touch the power and engineering of your physical body. It's precious, sacred, and supernatural machinery.

You're fearfully and wonderfully made, and you house His Spirit along with your soul.

It allows us to engage with the material environment. We do this with our five senses. We love to look at beautiful flowers, smell perfume, taste delicious food, hug our loved ones, or hear the ocean waves. Life is the greatest gift we have. And we experience it through our body.

Think of it like this, if you lent your computer to someone and they messed it up with coffee spills, marker stains, and missing keys, you'd be furious. When I understood how much damage I did to this divinely created machine, I felt convicted to honor it.

Our body is more valuable than any computer, car, home, or possession we'll ever own. It's the only home we live in our entire lives, it's our permanent earthly address.

As a vehicle or instrument it carries out good or evil. It can do what we want only, or it can do what God is leading us to do. The body can rule us with temptations and lusts. We've been there, done that.

As a result of it being a vehicle, we need to fuel it properly. Like a cell phone charger charges your cell phone, your body recharges with food, water, sleep, movement, affection, sunshine, and air.

If we don't breathe for three minutes, we die; if we don't drink water for a week, we die; and if we don't eat for a month (this is where body fat really comes in handy!), we die.

> **The most high-end Tesla can't touch the power and engineering of your physical body.**

Signs of Bondage in Body

- Can't say no to temptations that titillate your senses. My cookie story in the last chapter had its physiological aspects of bondage, because the brain was addicted to sugar, caffeine in the chocolate chips, and flour. I simply couldn't say no.

- Obsessed with how you look, extremely self-conscious, or negative about your face, body, or features.

For freedom, we'll master body care in upcoming chapters.

Soul – Emotions, Intellect, Volition (Will)

The soul is unique and so special the Christian faith is oriented around Jesus Christ who died and resurrected to save it.

We can't see the soul like we can the body, but our voice is evidence we exist.

Soul also means psyche, self, personality, or psychology.[4]

The blood, the red juice, carries the life of a person as in the DNA of the personality, interests, strengths, desires, weaknesses, character traits, and values that make a person fundamentally who he or she is—your identity.

Your soul has heart. To feel is difficult for most of us, but we need to get good at it. Because, health ailments may manifest in the body, but they've got soul roots. Psychologists call this somatization when a health issue manifests from emotional anxiety or an unresolved trauma.[5]

Henry W. Wright, author of *A More Excellent Way,* studied physical ailments from a spiritual and psychological perspective. He said, "The key roots behind disease are bitterness, accusation, occultism (witchcraft/satanism), envy, jealousy, rejection, unloving spirits, addictions, and fear."[6]

When negative emotions aren't resolved, we'll see dysfunctional patterns, such as addictions, broken relationships, and lack of professional and personal progress.

Our soul can be bound in emotional states, especially those that run through generations in our family, such as anger or grief.

Traumas, like verbal, physical, sexual, emotional abuse, or neglect, we experience as children can injure our soul. Injuries create soul wounds also called emotional wounds. And much of the time we emotionally eat because a soul wound was pushed.

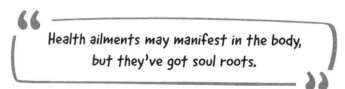

> **Health ailments may manifest in the body, but they've got soul roots.**

What's interesting is, no matter what you do you can't stop your baby boy from growing up into a man. But the emotional body can have its growth stunted at the time of the trauma, and it can stay stuck as a child in an adult body. It's called arrested development.

And now you've got your answer for why fifty-year-old people act fifteen.

Emotional wounds of the past pull on our present. And our soul's past affects our present weight and eating condition. When a binge happens, it's a signal that we've triggered an unresolved soul wound. We'll focus on this when we **Enact an Emotional Strength Training Plan** in Chapter 18.

Also note that the psychological needs of the soul are just as strong as the physiological needs of the body. These psychological needs are what holds in place our validation of our self-worth, for good or for harm. Bad habits reinforce a strong psychological need, despite the irrationality. We'll walk through these psychological factors in **Grubbology** (why we eat excess) and **Chubbology** (how excess weight keeps our soul safe).

Our intellect consists of mindsets, mentalities, value systems, and thought patterns. Your soul and mind are scientifically integrated with the body and brain.

Thoughts are words, and words carry the power of life and death. A healthy mind supports a healthy body. The mind is bound in the form of the dieter's mindset because it's a mindset that entraps us in poor health. We'll explore this in **Adopt the Freedom Mindset** in Chapter 17.

Volition is our soul's right to use our mind and emotions for our decisions. We get to choose. We can choose life or death with our choices.

We get to choose to grow, learn, change, heal and transform or stay stuck. I want to be free, how about you?

> " A healthy mind supports a healthy body. "

Signs of Bondage in Soul

- Emotions are difficult to identify or express
- Difficulty controlling emotions, emotionally reactive or driven
- Thinking distortions – all or nothing, negativity, unrealistic
- Past traumas, abuse, or neglect
- Easily triggered or offended
- Feeling followed by a dark cloud
- Self-sabotaging behaviors and choices

Soul Encouragement

God is the master chef. In His kitchen He makes souls with special sacred ingredients. He sprinkles in talents, strengths, and special experiences to shape you to find them. He bakes in His purpose for each soul. He puts heavenly spices in and infuses us with His love. What's amazing about His recipe is that no two are alike.

Each soul recipe is made once and only once. It cannot be duplicated. It's an expression of His Glory and of His master creativity. He makes each soul with joy to enjoy. You are special and loved.

Therefore, our best life requires demands us to be free. When we're in bondage to the soul, we're unable to love others because we can barely love who we are to be. And by the way, your body—your physical looks—are a part of that unique beauty.

You're created you the way you are for many reasons. A worthy soul is one that seeks to be a godly presence for others in humilty.

It's harmful to believe we're worthless.

Essentially low soul-worth, as evidenced by how we mis-care for our bodies, health, and souls, is in opposition to growth because insecurity and false humility creates self-focus, self-consciousness, and all-about-me attitudes, looking for validation and love in all the wrong places.

To be free, we choose to heal. Your desire to make a commitment to freedom from poor body care is a giant step in the right direction. There's amazing fruit from a restored soul.

Spirit – Conscience, Intuition, Communion

The Spirit is the breath of God and gives every living thing life. Think of Spirit as what causes animation. A cat or dog has life, as does a plant.

If it's born, lives, and dies, it has the spirit of life. The human spirit, however, is comprised of conscience, intuition (innate wisdom), and communion with the supernatural. It's the water.

Therefore, every person alive has a spirit that connects us with the supernatural. The difference in Christ lovers is Jesus imparts to us the Holy Spirit, the oil. The human spirit is life whereas the Holy Spirit can bring us truth. Also please feel free to use your own idea of spirit or God, but I will use Holy Spirit.

Our conscience helps us to discern between right or wrong. As children we tend to know when something feels right or wrong, this is our conscience at work. Conscience supports deeply embedded emotions, such as love, fear, shame, or guilt. It helps us to discern general human moral behavior—good from evil.

Intuition is our gut sense that helps us discern beyond the five senses of the body. Did you ever want to call a friend, but then suddenly she's calling you? This is your intuitive sense at work. Intuition is a sense of going the right direction. Let's allow listening to our intuition to guide positive choices. Another word for intuition is wisdom.

Your Spirit connects with the *spiritual realm*. Ideally, we commune with the Holy Spirit. However, a person can deal with spirits that aren't right. For example, the Bible mentions the Holy Spirit and also spirits, such as fear, jealousy, strife, and rebellion. But just look at the news. Have you seen it lately? Enough said. Some of our headlines are the working of a wrong spiritual connection.

Signs of Bondage in Spirit

- Strange creepy presence
- Legalistic or controlling
- Lack of fruit of the Spirit
- Carnally minded, worldly
- Perversity
- Sense of heaviness

Every human has a spiritual side to cultivate. Some religious folks aren't yet in touch with their spiritual side. I know this because some religious aren't loving or godly, as they come across as prideful, horribly judgmental, unkind, ungrateful, and shaming toward their own self and others. This self-righteous attitude comes from a soul insecurity like the need to be better than someone else because of low self-worth, not out of God's love for each person.

When we don't like the fruit, we must look at the roots. Weight struggles are a symptom. They're a manifestation or fruit of our body, soul, and spirit. We're always able to connect to spirit and cultivate the fruit of the Spirit because, like a healthy body, the fruit of the Spirit is already inside of us.

The fruit of the Spirit is love, joy, peace, longsuffering, kindness, goodness, faithfulness, gentleness, self-control. Against such there is no law.

As our soul heals, we manifest more fruit of the spirit. The way to freedom in body, soul, and spirit is to be led of the Spirit. The Holy Spirit is our divine connector and help.

> When we don't like the fruit, we must look at the roots. Weight struggles are a symptom. They're a manifestation or fruit of our body, soul, and spirit.

Let's learn to walk by the Spirit and not the flesh. You've got a foundation, it's time to get to work. Next up, we'll put together an action plan to overcome.

REFLECT & SHARE

1. Can you sense the differences between your soul, body, and spirit?

_____

_____

_____

_____

2. In what areas of your life are you walking by the Spirit?

_____

_____

_____

_____

3. In what areas of your life are you walking by the flesh?

_____

_____

_____

_____

• CHAPTER 5 •

THE CALL TO WEIGHT & EATING FREEDOM ACTION PLAN

Commitment is like a balloon. Apply a little pressure ...POP!

T he path to weight and eating freedom starts with our commitment to freedom. Freedom is the ability to exercise options, to choose, to be in control. But we often don't feel in control in weight or eating behaviors.

The way we gain freedom is to commit to freedom itself, not diets, crazy workouts, starvation, or temporary fixes—but freedom. Christ is our liberator. We're not to live in torment, temptation, or intemperance. We're to live transformed.

The Call to Weight & Eating Freedom Action Plan boosts your commitment to get through the hard conversations we'll need to have, and the real habit change you'll want to make, to enjoy a whole and free life. The journey isn't easy ahead. These five actions help build your

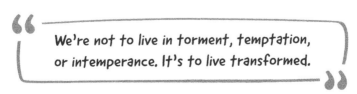

> **We're not to live in torment, temptation, or intemperance. It's to live transformed.**

commitment to freedom on days you'd prefer to retreat into a bag of denial. So, let's roll up our sleeves and get to work, shall we?

Action 1: Commit to Freedom

Let's acknowledge our truth: we don't want to change. A part of us likes to eat whatever greasy, fatty, crunchy, salty, or sugary food we can get our hands on.

I dream often, and one dream was telling. I was in a jail cell. A wide-open door stared back at me, but I remained on top of the plush bed, just looking at the door. Our lives are like this dream. We've been set free. Salvation has come. The door is open. But because we're so comfortable in our plush beds, we stay there, unwilling to pick up our beds and walk.

We don't know what to expect in our freedom.

To get out of bed, walk across the room, and out the door into the unknown is far scarier than lying in the comfort of what we know.

Jesus healed a man who had the same unconscious desire to stay stuck in the all too familiar bed. "Jesus said to him, 'Rise, take up your bed and walk'" (John 5:8). The man's obedience led him to freedom. It's not Jesus' desire for us to stay in bed—otherwise known as what's comfortable. We are to move and walk. Walk in love, walk by faith, walk in joy, walk in peace, walk on water. All of it requires action and a commitment to being free instead of bound.

Even though dieters make at least four attempts to lose weight each year, 90 to 95 percent of dieters regain weight.[1] This means the first, second, and third attempts weren't successful. Consider, all the times you've stopped and started a diet. Insanity is doing the same thing over and over again and expecting a different result. What if you stopped the temporary attempts altogether and committed to freedom instead?

Good news: freedom starts today. No more commitment to procrastination. You've already waited long enough for a weight loss miracle. It's not coming. Isn't that a relief? The miracle is your commitment to freedom.

Your freedom starts with your next bite—not when you're ready, not when you want to, but right now.

If you don't feel "ready," that's okay. Are you willing? Willingness and readiness are two different things. If you're willing, you'll soon be ready, but we're rarely ready without first being willing. Let's be bold and speak our commitment out loud.

Take Action: Speak Freedom Declarations

Take a few minutes to declare your willingness to **commit to freedom.** Words have the power of life and death, so use them to declare your personal freedom

Freedom Declarations: Say the following declarations out loud like you're rooting for your favorite sports team or seeing outlandish news reports:

> I make great food choices!
> I live healthfully one day at a time!
> I am healthy and fit!
> I am whole and free!
> I am enough!

These declarations set the stage to complete this material. What other declarations do you need to say aloud? Declare them often, especially when you feel tempted.

Action 2: Cultivate Desire

Why do you want to be free? It's a simple but oh-so-important question. Is it for yourself? Your kids? Favorite pants? We need to know why we want our freedom. As Lisa TerKeurst says in her book, *Made to Crave*, "we've got to *want to*" end the health struggles for good.[2]

Lasting weight release is a side effect of a strong commitment to freedom in body, soul, and spirit. What other side effects do you believe God has for you? Desire is a fertile farmland. We cultivate it with the

> " *How much has weight and eating bondage killed your joy, stolen your mind, and destroyed your health?* "

seeds of faith. Each seed is a pumpkin patch of possibility. Think long and deep about all you hope to gain from your commitment to your best life.

One way to strengthen your list of why you want to be free is to tap into your anger about what weight and eating torment has cost you over the years.

How much has weight and eating bondage killed your joy, stolen your mind, and destroyed your health? How many hours have you wasted thinking about this? How has this issue limited your career? How many events have you canceled because you felt too ashamed about your body size? How many times has low body esteem affected photo taking with your spouse or loved ones? We know we don't want the double chin, heart disease, diabetes, self-consciousness, or difficulty breathing, but what do you want?

Take Action: Create Your List of Reasons

Create a list of specific reasons you want to be healthy and free for life and win the weight and eating battle for good. Be unfiltered. List whatever your heart whispers. If animal print speedos pop up in your heart, don't judge or try to make it wrong or right, just jot it down.

You'll need to be real with yourself to stay motivated throughout the journey to weight and eating freedom. By the way, this won't be a list you set and forget.

This list will actively grow. Add to your list any reasons that come up as they pop up. And post your list somewhere you can be reminded of your reasons, like the refrigerator, car dashboard, or your desk. Be creative.

There're thousands of reasons to make a change in your health. List as many as you can. My list has more than 200 reasons. Reasons such as: I want to honor God in all things, be around for my children and their children, complete my divine assignments well, and easily bend down to pick something up.

Create your list by answering the following questions:

1. Why do I want to be free from weight and eating bondage? List as many reasons as possible.

2. What's my biggest reason to make a change? Put a star next to your biggest reason.

3. What do I want to gain from letting go of weight and eating struggles? Add to your list of reasons.

4. What don't I want any longer? Flip your answers from what you don't want to what you do want.

Action 3: See Your Vision

A vision motivates us. A good one excites us so much we run with it. As the vision of the life and health you desire sharpens, you increase your commitment and chances of success.

A powerful example of visualization is Dr. Martin Luther King, Jr's *I have a Dream* speech that reflects in America today.

To illustrate the scientific power of visualization, Guang Yue, an exercise psychologist from Cleveland Clinic Foundation in Ohio, compared "people who went to the gym with people who carried out virtual workouts in their heads."[3] While a thirty percent muscle increase was attained by those who went to the physical gym, a thirteen and a half percent increase was attained by those who did a mental workout.[4]

Don't use this as an excuse to eat donuts and imagine lifting weights in your head. Use it to complete the next action. Go ahead and design your promised land vision.

Take Action: Write Your Day in the Life Vision

Write your day in the life of your whole and free you vision. Use your list of desires to guide you. Think about an ideal day in your healthiest life. From the time you wake up to the time you retire at night, write out what you'd like to do, how you'd feel, what you'd eat, how you'd eat, and how you'd interact with the people around you. Use your creativity but write every detail out and be vivid.

> Possibility starts with imagination.

As a second option, if your vision feels as fuzzy as an old-school television station before cable, don't be discouraged. Just like with a wire hanger antenna, visions can be adjusted to sharpen them. Possibility starts with imagination.

Try to look at your life as though it were a page in a magazine. See yourself doing a healthy activity and decide what you're wearing and what emotions are expressed on your face. If you can't imagine yourself whole and free, it won't come to pass.

It was William Arthur Ward who said, "If you can imagine it, you can achieve it. If you can dream it, you can become it."[5] And Solomon who said, "For as he thinks in his heart, so *is* he" (Proverbs 23:7a). Write all about what you envision.

Action 4: Take 100 Percent Responsibility

Toddlers make messes other people clean up. But as mature adults we realize our rooms are messy because we made them messy. If we want it clean, it's our job. Responsibility is just that, cleaning up our mess.

The secret to freedom is that it's not free. Freedom requires our willingness to take ownership over our full self—body, soul, spirit, thoughts, emotions, actions, and choices—past, present, and future.

Your current condition isn't your spouse's fault, your children's fault, or God's fault. It's yours. Own it.

And as tempting as it is to blame the devil, genetics, the media, the food and drug industry, an underactive thyroid, or a demanding job, we're not going to allow anyone or anything to be responsible for our own choices but us.

We're taking our power back from all blame. This is how we gain momentum, hope, and more power to reach our goal. You are powerful so stop giving your power away.

> **We're not going to allow anyone or anything to be responsible for our own choices but us.**

Perhaps, the best way I found to take 100 percent responsibility was to walk through the twelve steps. When I learned about the steps, I realized this is the way we ought to be healing with God anyway.

Bill Wilson and Dr. Bob Smith discovered these steps when hopeless from alcohol. Bill, a successful broker, and Dr. Bob Smith, a physician, both damaged their lives with alcoholism.[6]

Alcoholics Anonymous is a successful tool in the journey of freedom for those with a drinking problem, as Celebrate Recovery, Overeaters Anonymous, Food Addicts Anonymous, and many other groups are also tools for those who have a weight and eating problem.

> **The twelve steps aren't for the weak, foolish, or struggling, they're for the strong, wise, and responsible.**

Bill was heavily inspired by the Bible, but he wanted to create a support group that allowed for freedom from alcoholism, attained through a relationship with God and others, over religious traditions. The twelve steps seemed to be a spiritual download, creating the path to growing one's relationship with God and others.

The twelve steps are a powerful tool in the journey to freedom. I strongly believe we should be doing them as a way of life. This book covers what's not covered in a twelve-step group for holistic transformation.

The twelve steps aren't for the weak, foolish, or struggling, they're for the strong, wise, and responsible. We take full responsibility when we practice the twelve steps as a way of life, stop making excuses, and take charge of our own insanity.

Work the twelve-step process: it's one of the most responsible, respected ways to do just that.

Take Action: Work the Twelve Steps

What are your answers to the following questions?

1. Do you admit you need God?
2. Do you believe God can help you fully overcome?
3. Do you give God permission to help you?
4. Do you know what your character flaws are?
5. Do you seek constant character improvement?
6. Do you admit mistakes and errors?
7. Do you pray for God's help to remove character flaws?
8. Do you ask God to remove your shortcomings as they come up?
9. Do you apologize when you mess up?
10. Do you monitor your morals daily?
11. Do you pray for God's will and lean on Him to carry it out?
12. Do you help others get free?

Did you answer *yes* to the above twelve questions? Each question above relates to the spiritual path and things we ought to be doing anyway as a way of life. They provide a way to take responsibility of our harmful issues.

Sit your pride in the corner and work the steps. You can review the questions above and put them into action or research a twelve-step group you'd like to attend. Most groups meet over the phone, online via webinar access, or in person locally. You'll gain connections and a safe environment to share with people who understand. To win, you must be willing to take full responsibility.

Action 5: Enroll Accountability

Humility to realize you don't have the power or ability to do this alone is a crucial step to freedom. Life provides people for us to be accountable to—a husband to his wife, a mother to her children, or a child to his parents. Just as churches have elders and the United States President has Congress, we also need accountability to keep our delusional human egos in check.

An accountability partner is granted permission to call you out on any wrong thinking or limiting behaviors to what you say you want.

According to the Association for Training and Development, the probability of completing a goal is 95 percent if you have an appointment with a specific person.

Get to your next level by enrolling an accountability partner. Doing it alone—well, you've been there, done that, and it's time for lasting change.

Take Action: Connect with an Accountability Partner

Get a sponsor, therapist, accountability partner, or group. Schedule consistent daily, weekly, bi-weekly, or monthly meetings with this person or group. Use one, a couple, or all four of the types of accountability partners mentioned below in your journey.

For accountability enroll:

1. **A professional you pay.** The most powerful results come from someone you pay. A secret weapon in reaching our next level is

hiring a therapist or a coach who, unlike our loving but fickle friends or family members, will show up because of the high motivator of cash, checks, and any other forms of payment.

Find a good therapist or accountability coach. Just as there are medical doctors for the heart, there are emotional doctors for the heart, too, called counselors, therapists, coaches, or psychologists. Hire a professional. But, if you're wondering, "How in the world will I pay for this and shop organic?!" No biggie. Enroll one of the freebies below. (No organic shopping required.)

2. **A sponsor from your twelve-step group.** A sponsor is a dedicated person who has been where you are. When you get into a twelve-step group, request a sponsor and someone will be willing to support your efforts to abstain from binge foods, diets, and overeating.

3. **A mentee you give advice to.** Who do you give the most advice to? Nothing puts steam under us more than the possibility of disappointing people who think we're saints. Asking a mentee for help not only qualifies you for a humility honor award, but also creates a higher chance of success in meeting your goals. Your integrity with the appropriate mentee, adult child, younger sibling, or dysfunctional friend creates wins. If this person is mature enough to follow through, give them a try.

4. **A support group of friends.** Birds of a feather flock together. A group of friends, colleagues, or, better yet, get the book course *Whole & Free Health* activated at your church. Chances are you aren't the only one in your circle who struggles with weight and eating.

Round up two or more people and meet for an hour once a week via phone conference, at the park, or in your home. Be sure you don't meet around food. We don't want to be counter-productive by meeting at Chubby's Grill or Fat Burger, for example.

Keep in mind, most people don't set goals to be free. They set goals to lose weight fast. Whatever you do, stay focused on freedom, not diets, agreed?

To request your accountability of choice, do so in humility. Say something like, "Accountability Partner, I've struggled with weight and eating for a long time, and I'm ready to change. I need your support as I read through *Whole & Free Health* and make small, meaningful changes over the next several months. I'm not looking for dieting advice here, but accountability. Would you support me as an accountability partner?"

With your accountability partner, set small attainable goals between appointments, such as: finish chapter 5, post on *www.thechubbychurch. com*, buy pants that fit my current size, pray, find supportive don't buy the bag of popcorn, or choose to eat green vegetables. If it helps your accountability partner, support her in something she may want to achieve, too.

Persist through the Lows

The struggle with weight and eating is a weary one. We start making progress at breakfast then eat our hearts out at

> " Thoughts of I quit, I give up, or this is too hard aren't part of a winning mindset. "

dinner. This up and down, back and forth pattern exhausts our motivation, and we lose belief in our own ability to win and in Spirit's ability to help us.

The struggle at times makes us feel like God's an ant compared to the almighty French fry, making us too discouraged to persist through the hard times. But when the going gets rough—and it will—we'll keep getting back up.

Thoughts of *I quit, I give up,* or *this is too hard* aren't part of a winning mindset. Our motivation is to be authentic believers who do whatever it takes to serve the King of kings, refusing to live in torment, temptation, and intemperance.

It's not a straight line from point A to point B. This journey in weight and otherwise will look a lot like the stock market. It's a daily process of working out our salvation with many peaks and valleys to find out why we've been hiding in excess weight.

> The heart of your motivation must be freedom.

Unlike that cabbage diet, in this journey failure doesn't exist. To give up is an operation of the flesh, not of the Spirit. If you feel like giving up, then you're normal, but your motivation still needs purification.

The heart of your motivation must be freedom. With a pure motive, we can't fail.

The road to freedom is also lifelong. When the weight releases, you'll need to strengthen your commitment to freedom even more because your mind will trick you with suggestions like, "I'm healed, so I can eat whatever I want," and the chains of bondage can tie you down again. To get through, continue to work these five actions steps.

Keep Going

You'll use your action plan to persist through the spiritual and emotional resistance and lean into the discomfort of your chubbology one page at a time, one day at a time, one bite at a time. But smile at yourself when you look in the mirror because your victory is on its way. And because you're cute.

Go to
www.jendayiharris.com
to download your free action plan.

BODY

• CHAPTER 6 •

MASTER BODY CARE

Chain #1 – Body Neglect

I didn't mean to, it was a snaccident.

Chronic diseases in America represent 90 percent of the $3.3 trillion in health care expenditures per year.[1] Obesity is $147 billion alone.[2] Not only are chronic diseases, such as diabetes, cancer, heart disease, and obesity, on the rise, but on average 40 percent of them are preventable and many reversable with diet and exercise.[3]

Furthermore, 117 million Americans are dealing with at least one chronic disease.[4] And worse, America's youngest generation is at risk of dying before their parents if we continue these trends.[5] Physical health is one thing, yet mental-emotional health is on the same trajectory.

One in five US adults are suffering mental illness.[6] And because of a lack of affordable solutions, professional helpers, and the stigma of mental illness, over 40 percent of mental illness goes untreated.[7, 8] Hence, our spiritual condition, evidenced by our health—mentally, emotionally, and physically, is due for an overhaul.

My passion about health started in early 2000. As a fast-food junkie, I was amongst many Americans who ate what I wanted without a thought that I had responsibility for my health or any influence on it. I was at the mercy of a doctor's opinion or my taste buds as I shared earlier. However, I came to the realization that food is our fuel. If we have the wrong fuel, it will reap havoc on all of the body's organs and systems. If you feed a dog chocolate, you'll quickly see how that's not the right fuel as evidenced by its extra repugnant output.

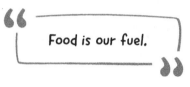

> **Food is our fuel.**

If you're sick and tired, you're losing the health battle because fatigue is a primary sign that your body's fuel sources aren't working.

The very nature of good fuel is to produce energy. If you find it difficult to stop snacking, get out of bed, play with your children, make love to your spouse, or walk up a few stairs, then you've got to be willing to upgrade your inputs.

Our fuel source affects our soul and spirit that are housed nowhere else but inside the body. And because the body is an interconnected, miraculous instrument, when one system is off, it affects another system and so on.

The statistics and research around the current condition of American health—physical, mental, and spiritual—is painful, grieving, and sickening. But there's always hope. No matter what your condition, the resiliency of the human body is incredible.

Body Care

We're not just a human body walking around. Our choices—what we eat, where we go, what we drink, what we watch, what we listen to, and what we do—matter in our body care.

Do you honor your body? To properly care for the body is to honor, respect, and appreciate it. It includes operating in self-respect and the respect for others in our sexuality, environment, clothing, hygiene, and physical needs.

We value, respect, and honor our physical body's needs by applying proper self-care. You may be out of touch with your physical body. You may not know when you're hungry or thirsty for water. You may not yet realize that you're eating because your exhausted or your dessert-like breakfast meal is causing your cravings for a midday coffee run.

As we move along, we'll discuss several triggers. We'll start with the body's *physiological triggers* because what may seem like emotional eating over sad feelings may be because the body's off balance chemically, since your body is a profound chemistry lab.

A dear friend of mine is a facilities manager of a church. His job is to make sure that the church is in good condition. To get the trash out, keep the bathrooms clean, take care of repairs, make sure it's protected from vandalism, and ensure the sanctuary's prepared for worship.

Just like a good facilities manager, we need to get and keep our sanctuary in order.

> **You are the sanctuary.**

The Chain of Body Neglect

Like car care, body care honors the vehicle that will fulfill our assignments in life, love our children, get to work, or cuddle with our pets.

We have the light of God, but it's not always glowing. We're so busy we rebel against good health by not making self-care a priority. We're overworking or overindulging on entertainment.

We neglect healthy habits and cause and create health problems. The American way of eating and drinking isn't working. And just because executives in high places are selling disease (packaged as edible deliciousness) doesn't mean we have to buy it.

You see, self-neglect screams, "I don't care about me! I'm unworthy of time and attention! I don't matter! I can't take care of myself! I can't manage my life!" Take care of yourself. It's selfish not to because, again, self-neglect leads to dependency on others and an inability to be there for others.

Body neglect is also a reflection of carnality. Carnality is being driven by the taste buds of the flesh more so than the needs of the body (organs, tissues, and systems). Most of the standard American diet isn't made by the sun and earth. It's made by machines inspired to addict carnally-minded consumers.

> Carnality is being driven by the taste buds of the flesh more so than the needs of the body.

To be carnally minded is death. The less discretion we have over what we eat or do with our bodies, the more evidence we're in our carnal, not spiritual, nature and driven by lust.

Our carnal nature puts a halt on God's transformative power in this area of our lives. I find I'm also not the most loving if I've overindulged or been neglectful of my body.

What about you?

BODY NEGLECT STRONGHOLD QUIZ

Put a check next to the answer that describes your body care and add the total points below. The higher the score, the more body neglect is present.

QUIZ

1. How often do you skip breakfast?

   ☐ (5) ALWAYS ☐ (4) OFTEN ☐ (3) SOMETIMES ☐ (2) RARELY ☐ (1) NEVER

2. How often do you drink half your body weight in ounces of water?

   ☐ (1) ALWAYS ☐ (2) OFTEN ☐ (3) SOMETIMES ☐ (4) RARELY ☐ (5) NEVER

3. How often do you cleanse your colon, liver, kidneys, or other organs?

   ☐ (1) BI-ANNUALLY ☐ (2) ANNUALLY ☐ (3) SOMETIMES ☐ (4) RARELY ☐ (5) NEVER

4. How often do you have gastrointestinal problems?

   ☐ (5) ALWAYS ☐ (4) OFTEN ☐ (3) SOMETIMES ☐ (2) RARELY ☐ (1) NEVER

5. How often do you exercise?

   ☐ (1) ALWAYS ☐ (2) OFTEN ☐ (3) SOMETIMES ☐ (4) RARELY ☐ (5) NEVER

6. How often do you take a multivitamin or supplementation?

   ☐ (1) ALWAYS ☐ (2) OFTEN ☐ (3) SOMETIMES ☐ (4) RARELY ☐ (5) NEVER

7. How often do you neglect your body when you're busy?

   ☐ (5) ALWAYS ☐ (4) OFTEN ☐ (3) SOMETIMES ☐ (2) RARELY ☐ (1) NEVER

8. How often do you sleep 7 to 9 hours per night?

   ☐ (1) ALWAYS ☐ (2) OFTEN ☐ (3) SOMETIMES ☐ (4) RARELY ☐ (5) NEVER

9. How often do you complain of being tired?

   ☐ (5) ALWAYS ☐ (4) OFTEN ☐ (3) SOMETIMES ☐ (2) RARELY ☐ (1) NEVER

10. How often do you get sick?

    ☐ (5) ALWAYS ☐ (4) OFTEN ☐ (3) SOMETIMES ☐ (2) RARELY ☐ (1) NEVER

Total Score:

Score Sheet
30–50 | You're in the right place!
20–30 | You've done some work and it shows!
10–20 | You're doing awesome!

_____

Focus on Habits

In the next several chapters, we'll focus on body habits for health correction because they're the easiest to correct and prevent. In order to improve weight and eating, we'll start with understanding our physical triggers.

A ***physiological trigger*** is caused by neglecting a biological need of your body. When triggered physically, we're vulnerable to overeat, emotionally eat, negatively obsess on body weight, shape, or size, and make other unwanted chubby choices.

We need the right habits in place to deter these triggers. There are six physiological triggers and six habits that we'll discuss.

The physiological triggers and their corresponding body habits are:

PHYSIOLOGICAL TRIGGER	BODY HABIT
Micronutrient Deficiency	#1 Nutrient Load
Toxic Overload	#2 Cleanse
Dehydration	#3 Hydrate
Poor Sleep	#4 Sleep
Inactivity	#5 Exercise
Hormonal Imbalance	#6 Balance

With all the talk on what to do with your health—take this prescription, do keto, do paleo, eat eggs, don't eat eggs, don't eat bananas, eat lots of bananas, eat this new superfood, drink wine, no, don't drink wine—it's confusing to figure out what to do.

It's been said the secrets of our future are hidden in our daily routine. Let's not continue to reject our souls' knowing: we must change our daily habits. Everyone who desires health has to habitize it. It's got to become who we are and part of our lifestyle. If you focus on the right habits, over time your health is guaranteed to transform.

We avoid confusion by focusing on the basics. The body habit basics bring the blessing. So, eat up the following chapters because the principles of the body habits will begin to work in you to create change.

Do so quickly so we can get to the really juicy soul section of the book.

Let's get to it.

REFLECT & SHARE

1. How have you neglected your body?

_____

2. How long have you procrastinated on making daily health a priority?

_____

3. Do you believe your treatment of your body influences you spiritually? How so?

_____

4. How have diets prevented you from adopting lifelong healthy habits?

_____

Note: All references to diabetes refer to type 2 diabetes, not type 1 diabetes.

Disclosure: Remember to consider all advice with a medical doctor. And the author and any affiliation with this book is not held liable for health recommendations.

CHAPTER 7

HABIT #1 NUTRIENT LOAD
AM I MALNOURISHED?

Physiological Trigger – Micronutrient Deficiency

Processed foods have eternal life without being saved or having ever been alive in the first place.

Experts point to fancy terms for the cause of excess weight such as inflammation, insulin resistance, or high glucose sensitivity. Yes, there's scientific proof of these things, and they matter. But why do we have inflammation, high insulin, or high glucose issues in the first place? Because on a daily basis we're eating processed foods and beverages loaded with chemicals and refined fats, sugars, flours, and salts causing *processed food addiction.*

Processed foods, stress-induced lifestyles, and environmental toxins are wreaking havoc on *all* of our body systems, making it more difficult to correct health, release weight, and eat better.

The one thing that seems to cure just about all major chronic diseases, according to books such as *The China Study*, *It Starts with Food*, and *The Micronutrient Miracle,* is quality nutrition. Friends, simply put, we've disobeyed nature's ideal food plan and we're paying the price.

The problem is deceptively obvious – ridiculous temptations from processed food addictions cause misalignment to how nature intended us to eat.

Micronutrient Deficiency Facts

1. Processed meats, such as bacon, hot dogs, salami, sausage, and lunch meats, can increase your risk of colon cancer by 18 percent, and raise the risk of pancreatic and prostate cancers.[1]

2. Americans buy and consume 60 percent of their dietary calories from highly processed foods.[2]

3. A minimum of 400,000 of the 600,000 annual deaths from heart disease are directly linked to poor diet.[3]

4. Deficiencies of vitamins A, D, K, B1, B3, B6, B12, folate, iodine, potassium, iron, magnesium, zinc, chromium, and manganese can contribute to mental instability and violent behavior.[4]

5. Genetic causes predict about 5 to 10 percent of cancers, whereas 90 to 95 percent of cancer is due to lifestyle, diet, and environmental factors.[5]

6. In a super study of 537,000 AARP members, those who ate red meat daily (pork, beef, lamb) had a 26 percent chance of dying from cancer, stroke, heart disease, respiratory disease, diabetes, infections, chronic kidney disease, or chronic liver disease during the sixteen-year study compared with those who ate it once per week.[6]

7. In the same AARP study, those who ate white meat daily (fish, chicken, and turkey) had a 25 percent lower risk of dying.[7]

8. Most Americans have low stomach acid levels due to a poor diet, which reduces nutrient absorption.[8]

9. Obesity and diabetes are linked to significant deficiencies in vitamin D, omega 3, chromium, magnesium, B3, B6, B7, B12, C, K, zinc, iodine, and iron.[9,10]

10. Plant-based eating heals heart disease, lung diseases, brain diseases, digestive cancers, diabetes, high blood pressure, liver diseases, blood cancers, kidney disease, breast cancer, suicidal depression, prostate cancer, and Parkinson's disease.[11]

> " *If you're a heathen and you eat well, you're going to live longer than you deserve based on this biblical eating principle.* "

The Great Physician, also our Master Nutritionist, said to eat all the green plant and seed-bearing vegetation (Genesis 1:29). In other words, eat foods rich in micronutrients. Micronutrients are amino acids, vitamins, minerals, and fatty acids that are the building blocks of the body.

We all know we should eat more fruits and vegetables and drink more water. And we know it deep inside our souls. Yet, we ignore that still small voice, until it becomes the doctor's voice who tells us we have cancer or congestive heart failure.

Sadly, on average, medical doctors receive about seven hours of nutritional education, but most barely get three hours.[12,13] So, they're ill prepared to recommend ways to help you heal with foods, only drugs.

Let's listen to America's favorite doc, Dr. Oz, who said, "Of all the personal choices you can make about your health, nothing holds greater influence than the food you eat. It has the power to fix your body, prevent some diseases, and even reverse others. Food is the extension cord that energizes and lengthens your life."[14]

If you're a heathen and you eat well, you're going to live longer than you deserve based on this biblical eating principle.

It's a fact that those who suffer from binge eating and/or obesity are malnourished.[15,16] Founding editor of the medical journal *Obesity Surgery* and Bariatric Surgeon, Dr. Mervyn Deitel said, "The commonest form of malnutrition in the western world is obesity."[17]

Nutrients are found in abundance in just about any fruit or vegetable. But they are rather scarce in engineered options.

Food giants that promote denatured, engineered processed foods and beverages.

Books like *Salt, Sugar, Fat* by Michael Moss, *Think & Eat Yourself Smart* by Dr. Caroline Leaf, and *Food Politics* by Marion Nestle explain the political landscape surrounding the food industry, and it's ugly. For now, we've got to learn how to eat better given the tantalizing environment we're in.

Micronutrient Deficiency Factors

Exploited Soil

Over the centuries, due to the exploitation of various pesticides and soil usage, we've seen dramatic changes in the quality of vitamin and mineral density in vegetables and fruits.

Nutrient density changes, as reported by the USDA, show that a tomato today has significantly less vitamin A, phosphorous, calcium, and other micronutrients than it did years ago.[18]

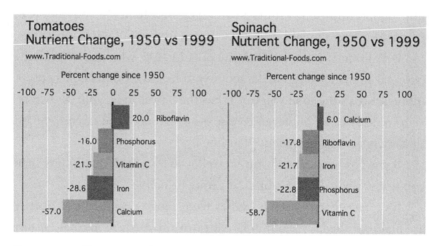

Figure 7.1   Tomatoes and spinach over a fifty-year period.

In the same timeframe researched, spinach shows a significant decrease in riboflavin, iron, and phosphorus, as well as more than a 50 percent decrease in vitamin C.[19] This means we need to eat more micro-nutrient rich foods to prevent diseases and heal, not less.

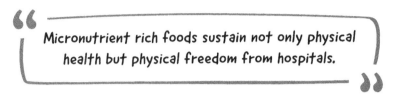

> Micronutrient rich foods sustain not only physical health but physical freedom from hospitals.

And those who are overweight or obese already have significant micronutrient deficiencies. In studies, over 55 percent struggled with iron deficiency (anemia) and more than 90 percent lacked vitamin D.[20] See fact #9 for other deficiencies researched. And the exact nutrients that are deficient in gastric bypass patients are the same nutrients it takes to digest food and the processed foods we're eating. Go figure.

A randomized Chinese study showed obese patients given a twenty-nine-ingredient multivitamin supplement over a twenty-six-week period improved their fat metabolism, reduced their body mass, and experienced better caloric absorption.[21] What are you waiting for? Take your vitamins.

Processed Foods and Meats

You, like me, may have grown up with French fries, ketchup, and over-cooked collard greens at holiday dinners as your only vegetables. The standard American diet creates micronutrient deficiencies.

Big food corporations hire talented food engineers who use lengthy formulas to create a bliss factor taste in processed foods.[22] This bliss formula calculates the exact combination of refined fat, salt, and sugar for us to become addicted to them.[23]

Therefore, when we eat processed foods, we don't get the micro-nutrients we need. And for our system to digest any food, we utilize nutrients. Micronutrient rich foods sustain not only physical health but physical freedom from hospitals. Deficiencies cause cravings and poor organ functioning, including brain issues like dementia.[24]

Surprisingly, when you get more micronutrient foods you can correct ailments to the tune of several prescriptions. In the documentary *What the Health*, an excellent watch exposing our morally twisted environment, two women experimented with a micronutrient rich eating plan.

Amy was burdened with her blood work, as she should've been because it revealed she could die of a heart attack any second. Amy's meds included heart pills, chronic pain pills, stress pills, muscle relaxer pills, and asthma pills. She had no energy, trouble walking, and couldn't breathe well. After two weeks of micronutrient rich foods, no meat, and no processed food, she eliminated all those pills.[25]

The same thing happened to Jane who had chronic arthritis in her hips. She used a walker to get around in her early sixties. She took six asthma medications, antidepressants, and more medications to manage their side effects.

After two weeks of nutrient dense plant foods, she walked normally, felt vibrant, and stopped her medications. Amy and Jane reversed disease through nature's instructions for what to eat most.[26] And weight and eating freedom was a side effect of their renewed health.

> "Any way you slice it, we're not meant to eat human-engineered foods in the amounts we do."

Not only does micronutrient deficiency drive up prescription bills, as a physiological trigger it causes cravings. Specific links to micronutrient deficiencies are found with various cravings.[27] For example, someone who lacks magnesium or iron may crave chocolate or coffee.

Due to deficiencies, cells become stubborn, toyless toddlers in a toy store, like *Bebes Kids* or *Children of the Corn*. When cells are in need, they'll take from other organs. Over time deficiencies create reduced capacity from our organs and systems. Seriously, it's scary to the neighboring organs to consistently lack nutrients, especially for the bones.

Any way you slice it, we're not meant to eat human-engineered foods in the amounts we do. Nutrient dense foods are plant-based foods with one word that describes their content, such as kale, spinach, apple, or onion.

Toxic foods have toxic ingredients you can't pronounce. A simple (yet complex) remedy is to commit to increase your ratio of real to processed foods. Think about it: how much of your daily intake is processed? Reduce that number and increase real foods.

Poor Digestion

Due to poor diet, evidenced by digestive issues such as diverticulitis, irritable bowel syndrome, gas, belching, stomach aches, or constipation, processed foods cause our intestines to have less than optimal absorption.

An estimated 74 percent of Americans have digestive health problems each month.[28] After a meal if you find yourself tired, bloated, or mitigating unwanted music that insists on coming out of your rear end, chances are your digestive health is off. To extract more nutrients out of your food, we'll need to practice digestive wellness.

Chew. Digestion starts well by chewing well. It's a simple free thing we can do to increase our nutrient absorption. Salvia is enzyme rich. When we chew well, there's less work for other organs. Do you eat fast? I used to be queen of fast eating. Once I ate a grapefruit and forgot I ate it because I ate it so fast. I spent at least fifteen minutes looking for it! Slow down to thirty chews per bite.

Churn. When food hits the stomach, it churns into chyme. According to Dr. Elizabeth Lipski who wrote *Digestive Wellness*, most Americans suffer from low stomach acid and don't know it.

Many symptoms exist, but a few are indigestion, bloating, brittle nails, leaky gut, or autoimmune disease. Low stomach acid throws off the endocrine system that's needed to regulate body weight and appetite related hormones.[29]

Stomach acid naturally reduces with age. But it's decreasing sooner due to our diets. When you eat a heavy meal consider betaine hydrochloride supplements or try apple cider vinegar in water to turn up the heat.

Synthesize. The liver and pancreas secrete digestive enzymes to break down foods. Processed foods and binge eating causes digestive enzymes to deplete.[30] We may not have enough lipase (breaks down fat), protease (breaks down protein), amylase (breaks down carbohydrate), and a host of other enzymes to synthesize what we consume.

In particular, we may have a stressed gallbladder or have no gallbladder at all. This tiny organ supports fat metabolism by secreting lipase and bile to break down fats.

I wore mine out when I ate whole sticks of butter … daily. As my Inner Glutton would say, *What's matzah without a heap of butter on top?* Digestive enzyme supplementation is essential to support absorption for those of us who have, up until now, overindulged on cheese, chocolate, and chips.

Utilize. The small intestines are a tremendous factory to distribute chyme into usable or non-usable raw materials that feed organs and systems.

Hippocrates, the father of modern medicine, said, "All disease starts in the gut."[31] And the more research I do, the more I see this truth.

Your gut is a strong influence on the whole body and talks to your brain.[32] Much of the body's neurotransmitters like serotonin, dopamine, and epinephrine are made in the gut. Our gut has an incredible field of insight in its enteric nervous system (ENS), which affects mental health and, consequently, emotional eating.[33]

Gut health is vital to micronutrient absorption. A few problems in the gut that are interrelated may be:

Leaky Gut (Intestinal Permeability)

Dr. Josh Axe's research shows that leaky gut is a leading cause of many health problems.[34] Symptoms include digestive problems, thyroid issues, bloating, and fatigue.[35]

With leaky gut, the digestive lining in the intestines leak toxins, bacteria, and other particles into the blood stream that typically would go through the small intestines for elimination.[36] It's causal to malnourishment.

Candida Overgrowth

Your gut—out of balance—may be what's behind intense cravings. Candida is a naturally occurring fungal yeast in the gut. When overgrown, it causes insatiable cravings.

Candida feeds off sugar (natural and artificial) and is exacerbated by refined fats, such as safflower, canola, or hydrogenated oils.[37]

A range of symptoms exist for overgrowth that includes yeast infections, bloating, psoriasis, eczema, and fungal nails.[38] Specific probiotics (healthy gut bacteria) help kick overgrown candida out of the gut house.

Small Intestinal Bacterial Overgrowth (SIBO)

The gut has three to five pounds of bacteria, in a ratio of about 15 percent streetwalkers to 85 percent happy housewives.

Now, we need streetwalkers, they keep us prayed up. But, if the bad bacteria in the gut universe take down the good bacteria's effectiveness, it doesn't look so good for the future generation.

Due to antibiotic use, low stomach acid, processed foods, and other factors, bacteria gets imbalanced, which impairs nutrient absorption.

A doctor can check total microbes (bacterial organisms). Under 103 organisms per mL is healthy, over 105 organisms per mL is considered overgrowth. Symptoms include diabetes, obesity, bloating, gas, fibromyalgia, pancreatitis, leaky gut, and candida overgrowth.[39]

Wheat Gluten

I must mention frankenwheat—a genetically altered version of wheat that is in baked goods, pizza dough, and pasta.[40] It's a featured ingredient in many processed foods.[41]

My friends, wheat isn't what it used to be six decades ago. Food manufacturers use frankenwheat or hybridized, genetically altered versions, because it binds to opiate receptors in the brain that cause appetite to increase.[42] It's addictive. This explained my cookie addiction, and it also explains your bread addiction.

All wheat isn't bad, in fact our body is made to digest it.[43] But refined, hybridized wheat and any other refined flour (even gluten-free versions) is asking for disease.

Author of *Wheat Belly*, Dr. William Davis, found that these new strands of wheat lead to leaky gut and over 200 medical conditions in the body.[44] Bottom line is our denatured wheat supply destroys the gut, our ability to absorb nutrients, and a healthy relationship with food.

Dr. Davis said, "The amazing thing about wheat elimination is that removing this food that triggers appetite and addictive behavior forges a brand-new relationship with food."[45]

But whole grains, including whole wheat, such as kamut or spelt, do have significant benefits to reduce disease, namely diabetes.[46] Do your best to reduce refined flours, find whole sprouted grain alternatives, or eliminate refined wheat flour altogether to reduce micronutrient deficiencies. We'll discuss this more in Book 2.

The best defense will always be a combination of micronutrient rich vegetables and fruits. They're loaded with fiber and probiotics to strengthen the body's ability to heal. Specifically, fermented foods, like miso soup, kimchee, or sauerkraut, support gut repair.

Heal with Food

We'll want to eat more living foods—foods that seed, grow, die, and decompose—to get our micronutrient health back on track. Living food brings life as opposed to dead foods like meats that putrefy, processed foods that seem to have eternal life without being saved, and vegetables once bright green turned black from overcooking.

A long shelf life isn't life. Most processed foods aren't beneficial at all—let alone in large amounts. They're tasty takers, not givers. Why wouldn't we choose life in all areas of our lives?

A balanced approach with substitutions works best. Switch from soda to club soda, from fried wings to baked wings, from candy bars to whole foods nutrition bars,

> **A balanced approach with substitutions works best.**

and from packaged items with ingredients you can't pronounce to packaged items you can pronounce.

Good nutrition mitigates cravings. In a healthy state, we want real nutrient dense foods, not junk food. While it's encouraged to research eating plans to increase your nutrition, don't obsess over diet fads. Keep it simple. Habitize body stewardship. On days you make eating mistakes or feel you've messed up, still nutrient load.

Everything is okay. There are no rules.

Create a (your name goes here) Eating Plan. A bio-individual eating plan is one that you create based on what works for your total wellness as far as foods, ingredients, and beverages. With a bio-individual approach, you honor your uniqueness and allow yourself to be more in tune with what your body, soul, and spirit need to thrive. Tap into your soul's quiet yet persistent desire to eat foods that nurture, restore, and heal.

Observe how what you consume impacts you. An ideal eating plan is one that decreases cravings, reduces negative emotions, and nourishes you at all levels. Eat the highest quality your budget can afford. Most of all, be led by the Spirit to reduce processed foods intake causing people everywhere to die before their time or to be really unhappy with their bodies while living.

> **An ideal eating plan is one that decreases cravings, reduces negative emotions, and nourishes you at all levels.**

Nutrient load in your meals. Add green vegetables to most dishes. I suppose a lettuce wrapped Snickers® bar may be too much of a leap, but eat mixed greens with meals or order spinach instead of the mac and cheese.

It's better to skip dinner than breakfast.[47] A quality breakfast is a habit that reduces chances of obesity and diabetes by 35 to 50 percent.[48] When someone tells me they're not hungry at breakfast, it's usually because they've binged the night before.

I think a nutritional start predicts a nutritional finish. In the morning, train yourself to nutrient load with a whole foods multivitamin (liquid, capsule, or gummy), omega 3 fat, fruits, and vegetables.

I mix things up with organic eggs (no yolks due to my butter damage) and kale, millet with fresh pineapple chunks and a green drink, juice a few bunches of celery, or blend a head of lettuce with kiwis, blueberries, and a scoop of plant protein. Mix it up. Food can be fun.

Tips to Habitize Nutrient Load

- Consider supplementation, such as B-complex, vitamin D, omega 3, whole foods multivitamin, digestive enzymes, pre and probiotics, and possibly betaine stomach acid for when you eat rich meals. I believe supplements now will reduce prescription pills later. For specific ways to heal your body, consider the reference guide: *Prescription for Nutritional Healing* for various supplementation protocols by Phyllis Balch, a certified nutritional consultant.

- Set small goals to increase green foods, such as eat three cups of green vegetables per day—the amount proven to ward off cancer.[49] A green smoothie in the morning makes it easy. Spinach, kale, collard greens, chard, romaine, celery, cilantro—the list is endless! Any of these options mixes wonderfully with fruit or a protein scoop. Green smoothie recipes are all over the internet, but JJ Smith leads the pack with her *Green Smoothies for Life* recipe book.

- Find ways to put living foods into each meal. Making spaghetti? Serve it on top of swiss chard. Like my green drink, there's plenty of twenty-first century ways to get your nutrition from companies that care about your health. Research a few.

- Keep learning. Learn about foods, organic living, or healthy cooking to support motivation and recipe knowledge. Attend nutrition related seminars or listen to podcasts. Definitely check out *What the Health* and *What's with Wheat* documentaries.

- Reduce inflammatory foods, such as cooking oils, sugar, flour, refined grains, processed foods, and cured meats. It helps to prepare your food at home and dine out less.

- Reduce television, it's correlated with obesity and diabetes.[50]

- Work one-on-one with a health coach or registered dietitian.

- Use a nutrition-focused food tracker. Chronometer, developed by physician and health researcher Dr. Joseph Mercola, is a wonderful way to track your nutrition intake to see what you need.

- Soak your grains and beans prior to cooking to reduce harmful digestive pectin on the outer shell for better digestion.

- Join me at *www.thechubbychurch.com.*

REFLECT & SHARE

1. How much processed foods did you consume in the last twenty four hours?

_____

_____

_____

_____

2. How many real foods did you consume in the last twenty four hours?

_____

_____

_____

_____

3. What tip can you implement right away to improve your real to processed food ratio?

_____

_____

_____

_____

CHAPTER 8

HABIT #2 CLEANSE
AM I TOXIC?

Physiological Trigger – Toxic Overload

The hardest workers you're in charge of are your organs.

Several weeks after I detoxed fast food out of my system, I tried Chinese food again. I played it safe with steamed chicken and vegetables with brown rice. It came with a sauce, and I figured a little couldn't hurt.

After my lunch, I ran the Cooper River in New Jersey. About a mile in, my lungs tightened, and I started to wheeze. I got halfway around the 3.8-mile bridged track and couldn't go any further.

Desperate for help, I tapped on the door of a highly suspect dude chilling in the middle of the day looking at the river in a tinted low rider. Got to love Jersey. Because I was in a medical emergency, I begged him to take me to my car.

I'll never forget when he dropped me off. With fear in his eyes he zoomed away like he just stole something. I got in my car, looked in the driver's side rearview mirror, and "Aaah! Sweet Jesus!" I retrieved my cell phone from the glove box to call my mother who lived closest to the scene.

Between strained breaths I said, "Call 911. I'm having an allergic reaction. I'll be right there."

My skin drooped, my lips enlarged by the second, and I turned various shades of red. Suddenly, my young twenty something fully detoxed hot self was now an eighty-year-old looking hot mess from the *Twilight Zone*.

I drove the five minutes to my mom's house, got out of the car, and crawled my way to the front lawn. The ambulance showed up right on time and the rest of the day was spent in the hospital with IVs of commercial grade Benadryl®.

The doctor insisted it was Monosodium Glutamate (MSG), a toxic ingredient in many Chinese foods, as well as processed and fast foods. In the past, I could tolerate chemical foods. I'd eaten them all the time. But after cleansing my body, I saw exactly which ingredients carried out a deathly attack against my system.

> **We need to detox on every level.**

I don't recommend being extreme like I was in my early twenties, but peek at the ingredients on any box you have lying around the house. From cleaning products, hair products, skin products, the office building, car exhausts, and electronic devices, toxins are everywhere. We're consuming things that are far from nature.

And our toxic environment is also toxic for us mentally, emotionally, and spiritually with so many violent and immoral acts on television. We need to detox on every level.

Toxic Overload Facts

1. Genetically Modified Organisms (GMOs) are in 95 percent of soy beans, 88 percent of corn, 95 percent of sugar beets, 90 percent of canola oil, and about 90 percent of all wheat grown in the U.S.[1]

2. In nine people tested, more than 249 toxins were found in each of them. Of those chemicals found, 147 are toxic and 76 are known cancer causers.[2]

3. There are over 3,000 chemicals in the processed foods arsenal.[3]

4. BPA (Bisphenol A) is a proven endocrine disrupter found in receipts, plastic materials, lined canned goods, and more. Those with higher BPA in urine were five pounds heavier than those with lower BPA in urine.[4]

5. Toxoplasma parasite infects 40 to 60 million Americans and is found in lamb, venison, and cat feces.[5,6]

6. Environmental Protection Agency (EPA) tests show more than 2,100 contaminants, including pesticides, heavy metals, radon, radioactive participles, and parasites in the tap water we drink.[7]

7. Children with the highest amount of pesticides in their blood stream are diagnosed twice as frequently with Attention Deficit Hyperactivity Disorder (ADHD).[8]

8. Glyphosate, an herbicide used in pesticide, is applied to all non-organic soil each year in the U.S., and it inhibits enzymes critical for body detoxification, healthy gut bacteria, and digestion.[9]

9. Wi-Fi, cell phones, and microwave ovens emit RF/MW electromagnetic radiation and studies not paid for by manufacturers found it can result in traumatic brain injury.[10]

10. Parabens, synthetic preservatives found in makeup, cough medicine, antidepressants, body lotion, and beverages, have been found in 99 percent of breast cancer tissues. Testing in 2,500 people found parabens in their urine samples.[11]

I know you thought your kids would be good workers for a family business, but the hardest workers you're in charge of are your organs! Our hardworking organs experience reduced capacity as we age. Most of this is due to the toxicity of the chemicals in foods we eat and drink, along with our environments.

Organs such as the liver, colon, lungs, and kidneys, as well as the spleen, have the task of filtering thousands of chemicals day in and day out. And to filter that many toxins is way beyond their daily job description in this millennium.

> **In this environment, our organs are working overtime to handle the toxic overload.**

For most of us, they've barely been able to clean up one job before another load hits the scene. In this environment, our organs are working overtime to handle the toxic overload.

Like our homes have functional operations and appliances so do our bodies. Imagine your toilet not being cleaned for a year. What about for several years? Your organs need to be cleansed, too.

When was the last time you cleaned your liver or colon?

In his book *Toxic Relief*, Dr. Don Colbert strongly urges us to cleanse our bodies from the myriad toxins we face every day. If our blood is toxic, we'll have all kinds of issues, like food cravings, edema, brain fog, and a host of illnesses.[12]

Three Areas to Clean Up

The Colon

First, we want to clean out the colon. Colon cancer is the second leading cancer in the United States and affects men and women almost equally.[13] The five foot long colon also has five segments and toxin-cleaning lymph nodes.

This thing has to work well.

If it doesn't, toxins clog our lymph system and recycle back into the bloodstream. Some toxins collect in the colon for decades. Most colon cancer patients are diagnosed after the age of fifty.[14] Emotionally, the colon is linked to bottled up hate.[15] And research shows about 42 million Americans are suffering from constipation.[16]

> **The less fiber in our diet, the filthier the colon is.**

Are you one of them?

To cleanse the colon regularly, eat more high fiber plant foods. The less fiber in our diet, the filthier the colon is. God designed us to need fiber and food to provide it.

High fiber consumption results in healthier body mass index, a healthy heart, and reduced cancer risks.[17] The recommended amount in America is 38 grams for men and 25 grams for women.[18] Most Americans eat 16 grams.[19] And years ago we ate 50 to 100 grams per day.[20]

If you don't have at least two bowel movements per day, your colon could be working harder for you. After all, how many meals do you eat per day?

Try black beans with 29 grams per cup, kale with 2.6 grams per cup, mangos with 6 grams per cup, and raspberries with 8 grams per cup, but not all together—that would be gross.

Healthy elimination is between twelve to twenty four hours after consumption.[21] You can check digestion speed by taking charcoal tablets. Track the time you take them until the time you see black stool.[22]

Besides adding more fiber into your daily diet, also consider a colon cleanser product. A good one takes a week for proper colon clean up. Don't be scared. You may imagine running to the restroom in khakis as you hold tight to your seat cheeks, but it'll be okay. Do a colon clean up on a stay-cation or work from home week to avoid loose stool fear. But hey, a little excitement in the office may spice up the work day.

Another thing I like to do, but it's not for everybody, is a colonic. I gave my seventy-something-year-old grandmother a gift of a colonic, and soon after she was zipping up and down the stairs. I was shocked. She leaped up those stairs like an African hyena. Prior to that she took f-o-r-e-v-e-r.

A colonic, also called colon hydrotherapy, is an enema process where several gallons of water are used to gently clean the rectum (the last part of the colon) which helps empty toxins.

You go to a colonic center, sit on a specialized toilet, and they fill your colon entrance up with warm water. They may sell you on more, but one or two should clean things up. Too much can stress the large intestinal lining, so it's not recommended.

Preparation for a colonoscopy is also a good cleanser, but it doesn't cleanse the colon adequately. The point here is to cleanse the colon on a regular basis, ideally with high fiber foods and a periodic cleansing program (quarterly to twice a year). Do whatever it takes to clean it up.

Harmful Organisms

Our blood carries all kinds of toxins, critters from fungus, molds, bacteria, genetically modified organisms (GMOs), viruses, and parasites. I'm going to emphasize parasites because they stimulate massive problems in health.

Most parasites get into our systems if we eat meat, drink tap water, eat sushi, have pets, or travel abroad. Dr. Hulda Clark, physiologist, has researched proof that "all illness comes from two causes, parasites and pollutants."[23] In her insightful book *The Cure for all Diseases*, she proves that parasites are a source of disease, including cancer, insomnia, asthma, diabetes, infertility, and HIV.

For example, diabetics are affected by pancreatic fluke worms in raw beef or cow's milk, called eurytrema.[24] Eurytrema can only live and multiply if wood alcohol is present in the pancreas.

Are you a cola drinker? Well, wood alcohol is found in most soda cans, water bottles, and packaged products. When the amount of wood alcohol elevates enough in your system and eurytrema is present, adult onset diabetes is birthed. This goes beyond what we learn around glucose-insulin levels, yet both need to be addressed.[25] However, medical doctors aren't as knowledgeable about the pollutant parasite factor.

I've had asthma since I was a child, but because I practice body habits, I haven't had to use my inhaler in years. Well, I noticed my breathing was rather troubled while writing this book. Of course, I took my inhaler, but it got worse.

> " Dr. Hulda Clark, physiologist, has researched proof that
> "all illness comes from two causes, parasites and pollutants. "

I ordered a parasite cleanse. After the first day of taking the cleanse, my lungs cleared up. Dr. Clark found ascaris parasites in her asthma cases, and Chinese researchers found the same.[26] Any parasite, but especially ascaris, can decrease nutritional absorption as well. As nasty as it is, parasite fluke worms get lodged in our organs.

Janelle, a participant in Whole & Free Health course, saw a nasty pool of parasites in the toilet after her parasite cleanse. This isn't something you'd tell your spouse about or anyone else for that matter. But no one was there to stop her excited surprise parasite party, so she told her husband. And against sexier spousal perceptions, she showed him. He admitted that he had passed the same. They were both parasite free. Anyone under your roof, including pets, could use a parasite cleanse.

To get rid of harmful organisms, certain herbs work miracles. Herbs like wormwood, cloves, and black walnut hull extra strength do an effective job killing them.

Dr. Clark has a great website that provides cleansing protocols and products. My miracle working parasite cleanse was from Global Healing Center. Whatever brand you choose, it should last six weeks to be most effective, which is the length of the parasite lifecycle. And like Janelle did, be sure to get your spouse on board with your detox adventures.

The Liver

The liver is a *Fortune* 50 company executive administrator (EA) to the CEO. It's where the blood is filtered for use. Like an EA would protect the CEO by filtering calls, meeting invites, vendors, and more, the liver's primary job is to filter toxins in the blood. Blood carries the lifeforce. And the liver transacts cellular metabolism with it that allows us to live our best life. Is it clean?

It's both a production factory and storage site for enzymes, hormones, vitamins, and minerals. It has approximately 2,000 chemical functions.[27] And amazingly, it can grow back up to two-thirds of its mass. We process about ten thousand pounds of toxins through the liver in a lifetime.

Like that toilet I mentioned, the liver uncleansed can get really congested. We know it's congested when we're fatigued or can't release weight despite efforts. It gets this way because we feed it drinks like soda and alcohol, and processed foods, which all create toxic by-products and slow functioning.

Other symptoms of liver congestion include low stomach acid, small intestinal bacterial overgrowth (SIBO), acne, gallstones, bloating, eczema, gout, psoriasis, diabetes, and autoimmune disease.[28]

The liver also gets congested with high fat consumption. You want to eat good quality fats. Find the best balance for fat intake for your body. The US government recommends 20 to 35 percent.[29]

The problem is we eat fast food or indulge in a five-layer chocolate cake for dessert, which is three days' worth of fat intake in just one sitting—food porn is real. And don't be deceived, deep fried anything, including French fries, are fat, not potatoes.

Fatty liver diagnosis began in 1980.[30] It's caused by a high fat diet. If we often indulge on chocolate, cheeses, meat, or high fructose corn syrup (which converts quickly to fat), we cause fat storage in the liver to overflow into the rest of the liver where it shouldn't be.

The liver must clean up the by-products of drugs, too—whether prescribed, over-the-counter, or otherwise. Medications are like getting a safety pin to close the frontside of your pants, while a split happens in the back. You take a pill to solve a problem, but you get other problems as a result.

> **"** Medications are like getting a safety pin to close the frontside of your pants, while a split happens in the back. **"**

It's reported that 70 percent of Americans take two medications and half of Americans are on at least two.[31] Medication, while beneficial in some way does have chemicals that cause toxicity and, hence, comes with a two paragraph list of possible side effects.

Anthony William is called the Medical Medium because of his spiritual gift into medical conditions since he was a child. In his book, *Liver Rescue*, he says, "Weight gain is really about the liver since there's no such thing as a fast or slow metabolism." He says that the two typical factors in weight gain—the thyroid and adrenals, which we'll cover in Habit 6—still relate to a sluggish liver.[32] It's about how fast or slow your liver functions, not metabolism.

This is good because Valerie in the Whole & Free Health course got her energy back and was able to release weight easier after her first liver cleanse. She used a liver cleanse program and did a liver flush.

A liver flush cleanses bile ducts in the liver. Typically, gallstones also get released in the process. Dr. Clark says, "Cleaning the liver bile ducts is the most powerful procedure that you can do to improve your body's health."[33]

A liver flush protocol involves taking a liver cleanse supplement, then using Epsom salts and olive oil to flush out stones. Ideally this is done twice a year. Before deciding on a liver flush think about your medical condition. You can use vegetables high in fiber to cleanse your liver instead. Focus on foods that heal the liver, such as dark green leafy vegetables, celery, apples, or squash. Emotionally the liver is the anger center. It harbors emotions of unresolved anger, resentment, and regret.[34]

Cleansing Protocol from Dr. Hulda Clark[35]

Dr. Hulda Clark recommends we start with a colon cleanse, then do a digestive candida cleanse per Habit 1, then the kidneys, liver, and heavy metals.[36] Heavy metals are a major source of toxic overload from old tooth filling mercury amalgams (from all that sugar), the environment, and mercury in fish.[37] Cadmium, used to make dentures, is five times as toxic as lead and correlated with high blood pressure.[37]

Look into a variety of cleansing systems and find one that resonates with you. It takes work, but it's worth it. A full system cleanse helps you to attain and manifest your weight and eating freedom.

Cleanse Flowchart
The following is a suggested sequence for those completing the full Dr. Clark cleanse protocol.

❶ Stay on the weekly Para Cleanse Maintenance Program until the 2-day Liver Flush. Do not take during the 2-day Flush. Continue after the Liver Flush is complete. A minimum of 4 weeks of the Maintenance Program is recommended.

❷ Repeat the 2-day Liver Flush 5 times. Wait 2 weeks between each Liver Flush.

Cleanse the Inside

Jesus gave a stern warning to religious leaders about looking good on the outside but not minding their character. He said, "Blind Pharisee, first cleanse the inside of the cup and dish, that the outside of them may be clean also" (Matthew 23:26).

While cleaning your body internally isn't the same as character, consider its principles. Some of us spend more money on clothes, makeup, shoes, suits, houses, or fancy cars to look good on the outside while our organs die inside. They're crying out for water, nutrients, and cleansing. And like Jesus's words to them, if we clean up the inside, it manifests on the outside. Be quick to clean it up.

Tips to Habitize Cleanse

- Schedule one to three full body cleanses per year. Scheduling your cleanse on the calendar will help you get it done.

- Get the junk out of your house. Remember it's not loving your children or your spouse to allow processed foods for daily consumption in your home. Despite what commercials portray, real love doesn't promote disease.

- Research cleansing products to support completing a cleanse in the near future.

- Consider Epsom salt baths, infrared or dry sauna visits, or exercise to assist in healthy detoxification.

- Use a loofah bar in the shower to stimulate your lymph glands to move toxics out. Brush under arms and behind knees.

- Fasting periodically is a great solution to cleanse for physical and spiritual reasons. We'll discuss this more in Habit 6, as well as in Book 2.

- Drink from a BPA free water bottle and decline receipts made with BPA.

- Try natural, one-ingredient oils to moisture your skin instead of chemical-laden lotions. Coconut, olive, or grapeseed oils work great for hair, skin, and nails.

- Deep breathe to pull the lymph system into activation and calm the nervous system.

- Join *www.thechubbychurch.com* to support your process. You'll also get ideas for products that have worked for others. And you can share any cleansing surprises without judgment.

REFLECT & SHARE

1. How do you think an internal cleanse will support your weight and eating freedom?

_____

_____

_____

_____

_____

2. What do you need to research in order to start a cleanse?

_____

_____

_____

_____

3. When will you commit to your next cleanse?

_____

_____

_____

_____

CHAPTER 9

HABIT #3 HYDRATE
AM I THIRSTY?

Physiological Trigger – Dehydration

It's better to have a pee dance than no pee dance at all.

Something most people don't know about me is that I'm a pee dancer. When I have to pee, I have to pee—now. Otherwise, I may dance in my pants.

As a professional speaker, I'm on my feet all day. I remember one time I needed to pee, and the class kept asking questions as I did my awkward pee dance. I darted to the rest room at the first break opportunity. When I came back in the room, embarrassed, I wanted to shout, "I'm okay! I didn't pee my pants!"

A friend, also a pee dancer, had me beat. At a campfire as stars glistened and the fire crackled, what started as an, "I'm laughing so hard that I'm crying," turned into, "I'm laughing so hard I just peed my pants!" In front of everyone, she shouted, "I'm peeing! Oh, my goodness, I'm peeing my pants!"

She quickly hovered to hold her privates, squirming every which way. Unable to stand upright, her face turned red and her smile transformed into a horrified O-like shape as she looked at the group. "It's running down my leg!" Someone ran over to give her a blanket to help her out. I wish I could say it was me.

No, I was with the other forty witnesses, hysterically laughing on the cold, dark, dirty benches stomping our feet in utter elation. But she was hydrated. Yes, ladies and gentlemen, she was hydrated.

Water drinkers are often inconvenienced by bathrooms. Yes, the inconvenience of relieving your body from its hard-working self to take two minutes to go to the rest room. What a pity.

Often, I pray, *God, please send me a restroom, quick*. Truly, I'm super grateful when I'm in a room that has a bathroom nearby. It lets me drink my water in peace, knowing I'll have a place to pee. *Aaah, the little things.*

> " It's better to have a pee dance than no pee dance at all. "

Your pee dance may not be fun in the moment. But, by golly, it's better to have a pee dance than no pee dance at all.

Dehydration Facts

1. We're made of 60 to 75 percent water. Our brains need 85 percent water to function, along with every other organ and function in the body from bones to eyes need water.[1]

2. Soda, energy drinks, and the like deplete your body of water causing dehydration because of high sugar and caffeine contents.[2]

3. Cancer cells survive in low-oxygen environments that are acidic. Water is the best, most cost effective way to increase oxygen to the blood flow.[3]

4. You get 20 percent of your daily hydration needs from fruits and vegetables that contain the highest quality water available.[4]

5. Light yellow urine and six to eight pee stops per day indicate we flush our systems well.[5]

6. In an eleven-year study of more than 190,000 people, one liter or less of water per day increased the risk of kidney stones by 75 to 86 percent.[6]

7. Water also hydrates the colon and supports healthy bowel function and elimination.[7]

8. Dehydration prevents sex hormone production, which is a primary cause of impotence and loss of libido.[8]

9. While not causal to stroke or dementia, one study showed that people who drank one diet drink per day were three times more likely to have a stroke or dementia.[9]

10. Dehydration causes toxic sediments to store in tissue space, fat, joints, kidneys, liver, brain, and skin. Water clears toxins.[10]

To survive we don't need as much water, but to thrive in health we do. I agree that it's not always fun finding a restroom when you're on the road, on a plane, or at the store. But body neglectors won't hydrate at the cost of inconvenience. That cost may be higher than you want to pay.

Cells are like sand—too many to measure. Each one needs H2O. In, *Your Body's Many Cries for Water*, Dr. F. Batmanghelidj—we'll call him Dr. B—shares incredible research on the impact of dehydration on health.

He attributes a lack of water to several physical concerns which include obesity, asthma, cancer, high cholesterol, insomnia, ADD, over-eating, hormonal imbalance, anxiety, pain, allergies, Alzheimer's disease, depression, high blood pressure, and arthritis.[11]

That's a mouthful.

He believed physicians should first recommend hydration therapy to their ailing patients. In his research proved by thousands of testimonials, it's evident most diseases stem from a chronic case of dehydration at the genesis.

Are you dehydrated? Besides the issues mentioned, other signs of dehydration are thirst, constipation, dry eyes, dizziness, poor concentration, joint pain, dry scalp, confusion, down mood, unexplained hunger, headaches, excess saliva, dry skin, or dry mouth.

We know we're hydrated when we show no symptoms and urinate about 800 to 2000 mL a day (3.38 to 8.4 cups) or have six to eight pee stops of urine that's light yellow in color.

Blood plasma is the part of the red blood cell that carries raw material for use. About 90 percent of it is water.[12]

For example, that plasma water goes to places such as the brain to make sleep hormone melatonin or the good mood neurotransmitter serotonin. Melatonin and serotonin, as well as many other hormones and neurotransmitters, are dependent on hydrogen and oxygen molecules of H_2O atoms for their chemical composition.

Dr. B in his book *Obesity, Cancer, Depression: Their Common Cause & Natural Cure* said, "The brain's need for water is constant and urgent."[13]

Per Habit 2, every day of inadequate hydration is toxin multiplication. The less hydration the more toxins get lodged in various places in the body. As babies, our bodies were about 75 percent water, and by old age it's about 50 percent.[14] Health declines mid to late life when we're severely dehydrated. Most cancers are diagnosed after age fifty.[15] Coincidence? I think not.

Dr. B calls high blood pressure a "gross body water deficiency."[16] Because groups of capillaries in the vascular system begin to go out of business until they get the water funds they need to reopen, blood pressure increases.[17]

> " The less hydration the more toxins get lodged in various places in the body. "

One in three Americans have high blood pressure.[18] Dr. B is also adamant about the brain going from a grape to a raisin in diseases like Alzheimer's as a result of hydration deficit.

Orthopedic Surgeon, Dr. Lorraine Day, had a breast cancer tumor that grew at lightning speed. She saw death taking over her chest. No matter what she did, it grew as big as a cantaloupe.

Days before she thought she'd die, she found Dr. B's book *Your Body's Many Cries for Water*. Hydration shrank the tumor in weeks. She blamed her excessive coffee drinking for her malignant tumor.[19]

Russell had "chronic unintentional dehydration" like many others.[20] He did the recommended water cure from Dr. B's suggestions, along with a home water filtration system. In two weeks flat he cured both anxiety and depression. How's that for an inexpensive prescription bill?[21]

Why We're So Thirsty

Everyday Water Demand

Our bodies are like a Big Gulp®. And each one of our trillions of cells has to take a sip.[22] This makes water the most in-demand substance in our bodies. We lose water every time we sleep (perspiration and breathing vapor), eat (water is used in the digestive process), or move (perspiration). Water needs also increase if you exercise, live in high altitude like me (Colorado), or live in a hot climate where you sweat more.

We need to replenish water on a daily basis, but once the day is gone, you can't get it back. Like sleep, each new day is an opportunity to make sure to fill your body's cup.

Too Many Options

Another problem is we're drinking soda, sugar-sweetened beverages (SSBs), coffee, and alcohol. Each has a diuretic effect, especially caffeinated drinks and alcohol. It's a good practice to drink a cup of water for every cup of caffeinated beverage.

Alcohol is also a diuretic, for every 2 ounces of alcohol consumption (the size of a shot glass) diuretic hormones activate and excrete 200 mL of urine.[23]

If you don't drink alcohol, do you drink soda? Americans drink roughly twelve cans of soda per week or about 38 gallons of soda each year.[24] Sugary drink consumption, especially sodas, increase one's chance of obesity by 27 percent.[25] And one can per day increases diabetes risk by 18 percent.[26]

Furthermore, 4-Mel is a known chemical ingredient in darker sodas that helps to caramelize their texture and is a proven cancer catalyst.[27] Like cigarettes, I believe these drinks should come with a warning label.

On the flipside, one can release twenty-five pounds a year just from replacing sugary drinks with water.[28] Given that diabetes is the seventh leading cause of death in the United States and cancer the second, it may be a good idea to pass on the cola or sweet tea.[29]

We're super blessed to have drinkable water available to us. Water drinking is a habit that must be a daily focus, and we're blessed because there's little cost to do so.

> **These signals can be confusing to an overeater because he or she will eat solid food when water was what was needed.**

Medications

It's no secret medication causes the most chronic dehydration symptom, dry mouth. Medications require more water intake than average. It's sad to see how many prescriptions are filled that cause dehydration for diseases and ailments that may have been a by-product of dehydration masked in other names. If not treated properly with adequate water intake you'll be hooked on high cost prescriptions for life because the first issue wasn't properly treated.

Mixed Signals

The physiological trigger of dehydration is one because the brain gets energy from either hydroelectricity (energy by cellular water) or glucose.[30] This is a major problem leading to weight and eating bondage because the executive pre-frontal cortex in the brain sends signals for water or sugar based on its needs.

These signals can be confusing to an overeater because he or she will eat solid food when water was what was needed.[31] If you drink water before eating food, you'll be able to better discern when you need food or water. And if you just ate within an hour or so, chances are you need water, not food.

Several testimonials from Dr. B's water cure involve men and women releasing over thirty pounds or more from drinking the recommended amount of water with a tiny bit of high-quality salt on the tongue every few liters.[32]

Water was the beverage of choice for humans prior to hundred million-dollar marketing campaigns for soft drinks. If you want to win the weight and eating battle for good, you'll want to trade your sweet cancer-causing sodas, warm cup of joe, good times alcohol, and energy drinks for good old fashioned H_2O.[33]

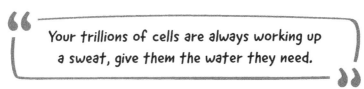

> Your trillions of cells are always working up
> a sweat, give them the water they need.

Solve Dehydration

Water is the primary source of energy. When fatigued or foggy headed, a tall glass of water is the first line of defense. Sources that dehydrate like an energy drink, should be the last. Your trillions of cells are always working up a sweat, give them the water they need.

The optimal amount of water to drink is not eight cups but much higher. The National Academies of Sciences, Engineering, and Medicine recommend 15.5 cups (3.7 liters) for men and 11.5 cups (2.7 liters) for women.[34] Dr. B recommends a half an ounce of water per pound of body weight.[35] But depending on your lifestyle, drink the amount that seems to work best for you.

Grab a Calculator to Figure Out Your Ideal Amount of Water Consumption
Total ounces = Your weight x .5
[Divide by 8 ounces to figure out how many cups you need per day]

Start today, drink your body's specific needs.[36] Also replace table salt with Himalayan pink salt or another high-quality unrefined sea salt of choice to get a greater spectrum of nutrients, which is vital in the body's water regulation process. Not much, but a little salt in your intake has many positive functions including opening up blood flow according to Dr. B.[37]

The best thing you can do as far as water quality is to get an in-home filtration system. A filter of some sort is necessary for tap water. Don't be a water snob, but just do what you can and follow all the habits to maximize effectiveness.

Whatever temperature water you drink is fine. Cold water is perfect for people who exercise or get a lot of activity. Hot water is great before, during, or after a meal to support digestion. Room temperature works well before a meal to increase fullness.

Dr. B recommends that we drink two cups about thirty minutes before meals and two cups every couple of hours after meals, but don't be legalistic about it. I sit a jug at my desk, pop lemon and straw in a glass, and pour and chug all day. It's better to drink up as much as you remember during the day so that you're not up at night interrupting sleep doing a horizontal pee dance.

> Carry your water bottle around like you do your cell phone.

All this to say, carry your water bottle around like you do your cell phone. Water will help you to curb cravings. And you'll get used to hourly or bi-hourly bathroom visits.

If the worst that can happen to you is a couple moments of the pee dance from time to time as you wait for the bathroom at a gas station, so what? At least you won't pee your pants in front of forty onlookers, right?

Tips to Habitize Hydration

- Carry your water bottle around like you do your cell phone. Keep water by your bed and at your desk.

- Drink as little as you can from plastic bottles but instead get a large, BPA/toxin-free plastic water bottle with a built-in straw. Replace all soft drinks with water. Reserve soft drinks for rare special occasions.

- Drink at least sixteen ounces first thing in the morning. Add lemon for more cleansing effects.

- To find out what your cellular hydration looks like, some fitness or natural health centers offer a body composition analysis. Try one.

- Eliminate caffeine and alcohol from your beverage options.

- Add flavor aids like fresh lemons, oranges, cucumbers or mint leaves, or flavor packets with no or low sugar.

- Set an alarm on your cell phone for every ninety minutes that reminds you to drink water.

- Take ten sips every time you do sip water. (Tip from a Whole & Free Health course participant.)

- Consider a reverse osmosis home filtration system to block up to 99 percent of toxins in the water supply.

- Read *Your Body's Many Cries for Water or Obesity, Cancer, Depression: Their Common Cause & Natural Cure* by Dr. F. Batmanghelidj, MD.

REFLECT & SHARE

1. Which tip will you try to support your water intake?

   _____

   _____

2. What beverages have you consumed in the past twenty four hours?

   _____

   _____

3. How can you replace your current beverages with water to support your health?

   _____

   _____

• CHAPTER 10 •

HABIT #4 SLEEP
AM I TIRED?

Physiological Trigger – Poor Sleep

*We seek out junk food when tired as
though taken over by the sugar demon.*

Lack of sleep is the root of all evil—evil attitudes that is. We don't realize how much we take a lack of sleep out on our waistlines or loved ones. We've all nodded off a time or ten at church. But maybe your pastor isn't all that boring. Perhaps your nodding off was just a sign that you're sleep deprived—along with other symptoms, such as road rage, snappiness, and overeating.

Some people have the spiritual gift of sleep, but that isn't me.

I've struggled with sleep in Colorado's dry climate. So, I've had to learn all of these ideas

> **Lack of sleep
> is the root of
> all evil attitudes**

from my own sleep changes. And sleep is similar to weight and eating issues because there's multiple factors that contribute to the quality and quantity of it. But the body habits help the most.

If you're like me, you may just like to stay up late in what researchers call intentional sleep deprivation. Only, burning the midnight oil on a consistent basis is detrimental to our health. We'll do our part to master the habit of quality sleep, which is seven to eight hours on a frequent basis. Note some people need up to nine hours for sleep quality.

Poor Sleep Facts

1. Less than six hours a night of sleep increases the likelihood of diabetes by 30 percent.[1]

2. Short sleepers are three times more likely to get a cold than eight hour sleepers.[2]

3. The gut produces 95 percent of serotonin and hormones that affect sleep. When gut balance is off, it can create chronic insomnia.[3]

4. Inadequate sleep causes hormonal changes that lead to overeating, slow metabolism, higher insulin resistance, and larger BMI (Body Mass Index).[4]

5. Blue light from cell phones, laptops, televisions, and other devices influence lesser quality and sleep duration if not shut off at least two to three hours before bed time.[5]

6. Partial sleep deprivation led to eating 385 extra calories per day.[6]

7. The largest body mass index is associated with less than five hours of sleep on average. Obese persons are likely to sleep less than seven hours per night.[7]

8. About 47.5 percent of obese short sleepers suffered sleep complaints compared with 25.5 percent of non-obese individuals in a study of 1,300 people.[8]

9. Psychological disturbances of hypochondriasis, depression, and hysteria are associated with obese short sleepers at higher rates than non-obese short sleepers.[9]

10. Alcohol may cause some women to fall asleep faster, but research shows they don't sleep as deeply through the night and have depressive moods.[10]

Wouldn't it be strange not to know you got to work until you were leaving? Sleep is one of those mysteries in life. You don't even know you've had it until you wake up from it. Sleep has two major functions. One is to clean up the brain and the other is to process the day's memories.

Your brain is a computer, sleep is the charge.

Adequate sleep happens in two main phases. Non-Rapid Eye Movement (NREM), which surveils the world around us so we're safe and Rapid Eye Movement (REM), the deep sleep, which puts us in a state of paralysis to not act out our dreams.

These phases ebb and flow in their five stages over about four to five cycles per night. Ideally, our brains move through the cycles over seven to eight hours. If it does, we wake up beating our chest with enthusiasm to take on the world. Isn't God miraculous to build in a process to do all of these things?

> Your brain is a computer, sleepis the charge.

The Case for Sleep

Poor sleepers don't fall or stay asleep smoothly, nor do they get enough sleep. Sleep apnea, snoring, insomnia, and short sleep are signs of an underlying health condition. Research confirms poor sleep or insomnia causes cognitive decline, difficultly learning, poor memory, bigger waistlines, accidents, and errors.[11]

On the note of accidents, drowsy drivers are the cause of 17 percent of fatal car accidents.[12] Not only is sleep deprivation while driving a horrible idea, poor sleep while we attempt to improve health is tragic.

Eve Van Cauter, Professor of Medicine at the University of Chicago called poor sleep the "royal route to obesity."[13]

We're setting a new route.

Americans slept more in the past year or two.[14] But about 30 percent of

> Poor sleep while we attempt to improve health is tragic.

us get less than five hours of sleep per night.[15] Most sleep less than six hours a night, which is 20 percent less than twenty years ago.[16] Research shows that being awake for eighteen hours affects the brain like a blood alcohol level of .08 to 1. Folks, that's DUI worthy.[17]

Shawn Stevenson, host of the podcast *The Model Health Show* suggests several tips for healthy sleep in his fantastic book *Sleep Smarter*. He said, "If you're focused on cutting calories to lose weight, then you might as well go ahead and buy yourself bigger clothes right now."[18]

Sleep is the bigger picture for weight and eating freedom. In particular, obesity and weight gain are attributed to less than seven hours of sleep per night.[19] Short sleep (less than seven hours within a twenty four hour period) can happen easily in what researchers call work week sleep debt. Those who slept an average of less than seven hours a night each week due to work had a 72 percent likelihood of obesity.[20]

And an even higher body mass index is correlated with less than five hours of sleep per night.[21] Research showed that people who got less than five hours were 29 percent more likely to gain about thirty pounds over the next decade and a half than those who slept at least seven hours.[22]

When tired, we eat more. When we lack sleep, the hunger satiation hormone leptin, which tells you not to eat, decreases by about 15.5 percent while the appetite hunger hormone ghrelin, which tells you to eat, increases by 14.9 percent.[23]

> We seek out junk food when we're tired as though taken over by the sugar demon.

This explains poor sleep as a physiological trigger. We seek out junk food when we're tired as though taken over by the sugar demon. We eat 300 to 550 more calories following a night of inadequate sleep quantity or quality.[24]

I've heard it called *tungry* (tired and hungry), which can make one *hangry* (hungry and angry). Studies also show our executive brain function that helps us with impulse control is compromised by poor sleep.[25]

Poor sleep equates to poor choices.

Let me emphasize this point a bit. We need sleep to rejuvenate our energy. When we don't sleep well, we're vulnerable to eating for energy. When we eat for energy, we choose energy dense foods—what's energy? Calories. Carrots are nutrient dense but not as energy dense (caloric) as candy.

And while the crackers, coffee, or candy bar seem like a quick fix, it's like duct tape on a car door: you'll need to keep taping it up to stay shut. Sleep quality and quantity patterns mimic poor eating choices.

Oftentimes we see exercise as the hallmark to better health, but sleep is just as important. In one study of two groups who ate well but one group exercised and the other group slept, both groups lost fifteen pounds.[26] So, if you eat well and sleep well, you're in for great benefits, including weight release, just as much as if you ate well and exercised. This is probably the best news you've heard all day if you're a couch potato. Soak it in, you actually don't have to exercise for health benefits.

But be careful not to oversleep either. Under sleepers increase cardiovascular risk by 11 percent, but over sleepers (more than nine hours consistently) are at a 33 percent increased risk of heart disease.[27]

Poor sleep equates to poor choices.

Sleep is the ultimate fuel to productivity, mental clarity, and good moods. Please, don't make bedtime an option. It's non-negotiable in the pursuit of health.

A Few Reasons for Poor Sleep

Toxic Overload

Toxic overload does affect our sleep. Toxic overload makes every system stressed in your body, including the brain's ability to fall and stay asleep. Dehydration plays a part here as well because the less hydrated one is then the more toxins multiply.

Dr. Hulda Clark tested high ammonia levels in the brain of those with insomnia.[28] Ammonia is a by-product of the metabolic breakdown of foods, especially processed ones and proteins.[29] In addition, ammonia levels paired with certain parasites create disease.[30]

There are a few amino acids Dr. Hulda Clark mentions that support the body's natural detoxification of ammonia. Namely, arginine, ornithine, and tryptophan.

Another piece to the toxic overload puzzle is high levels of histamine that affect sleep. We eat many allergenic foods, such as wheat gluten, dairy, soy, and peanuts, that processed food companies know are allergens.[31] Allergens can create addictions to the foods that raise histamine, a neurotransmitter.[32]

High histamine levels affect sleep. This is why antihistamines like Benadryl˚ typically put us to sleep. Per Habit 1, gut health is related to good sleep. A healthy gut will support healthy histamine metabolism to keep levels at bay.

With all the toxin overloads from daily life pollutants, processed foods, and such as discussed in previous habits, the sleep hormone melatonin gets depleted.[33] Besides sleep, one of melatonin's other functions is to rid the body of free radicals, making it an effective anti-cancer agent.[34]

In Chinese medicine, the circadian rhythm is also in sync with organs. Type something like "Chinese circadian organ clock" in a search engine for images of organs that are associated with specific times your sleep is interrupted. It may be a specific organ is congested.

For example, if you wake up between one o'clock and two o'clock in the morning, your liver is probably congested and overactive. Chinese medicine usually heals whereas western medicine, although I appreciate it, chops off or prescribes.

High Cortisol Levels

Cortisol, a stress hormone produced in the adrenal glands, is a strong determinant for rejuvenating sleep. Cortisol works in cycles, and it's supposed to be high in the morning for get-up-and-go and lower at night to relax into sleep. It works in the natural body cycle called the circadian rhythm.[35]

High cortisol happens whenever we feel anxious, are stressed, or eat sugary foods. Dr. Pauline Harding, MD says, "A single late meal, skipped meal, or high glycemic snack will raise cortisol at night and disrupt sleep."[36]

The body's ability to handle sugary, starchy flour products like pizza, potatoes, rice, bread, cupcakes, or pasta gets worse as the day progresses.[37]

> "A single night of missed sleep can raise cortisol by 100 percent."

High sugar, low fiber food choices increase cortisol for five hours following consumption.[38] Insulin increases are higher after eating for those who are overweight and obese, and so is cortisol.[39] A single night of missed sleep can raise cortisol by 100 percent.[40] Elevated midnight cortisol increases the risk for breast cancer.[41]

In Habit 1, I touched on grains and the gut, but non-sprouted grains are difficult on the gut because of the grain's shell. These grains secrete excess cortisol into your intestinal tract.[42] To support balanced cortisol levels, use sprouted grains (grains that are soaked prior to cooking).

Eat earlier and adopt more low sugar, high fiber foods to better relax into sleep. For us food addicts this is easier said than done, but promise you'll work on it.

There are many things you can do to balance your cortisol. The adrenal glands, the home of cortisol production, are one of the highest utilizers of vitamin C.[43] To balance cortisol, consider increasing vitamin C with broccoli, cabbage, spinach, or kale.

Magnesium also helps us metabolize food and sleep better.[44,45] Foods rich in magnesium are spinach, halibut, black beans, and pumpkin seeds. High stress cortisol depresses the immune system making us prone to infection".[46] This is why poor sleep makes us susceptible to colds and sickness.[47]

Caffeine is a deterrent to restorative sleep as well as to hormonal balance. A tiny amount increases cortisol, insulin, and other stress hormones.[48] It's best not to drink any at all, but you can drink decaf, drink black (no sugar which makes things worse), have seldom, or drink early in your day to reduce sleep problems.

Coffee has benefits but quality sleep, lasting energy, or hormonal balance are not one of them. Alcohol is also problematic for cortisol reduction and deep sleep. Refrain from alcohol on most nights or enjoy only on special occasions.

Poor Sleep Hygiene

Dr. Vyga Kaufmann, a psychologist in my neck of the woods (Colorado), has had success in her Cognitive Behavioral Therapy practice in treating insomniac clients with behavioral adjustments, such as using the bedroom only for sleep, making love, or reading a hard-copy book. She says, "Healthy sleep is shaped by the things we do all day."[49]

For example, if we work in the bedroom, where we should be sleeping, it will affect our ability to relax. I admit, I'm guilty of this at least twice a month, so I'm with you in efforts to reduce bad bedroom habits like spooning with the laptop.

Sleep hygiene describes protocols to set your bedroom up for successful sleep. It encompasses blackout curtains and removing screens, which include television, cell phones, electronic note pads, or computers from your bedroom.

> Reduce bad bedroom habits like spooning with the laptop.

Other bedroom oasis recommendations experts suggest are skin tone or neutral colored walls, high quality cotton sheets, a humidifier, *Fung Shui*, and green plants. Shawn Stevenson has the best sleep power tips in his *Sleep Smarter* book.

Artificial Lighting

Humans used moonlight, lanterns, and candles to enjoy the evening for centuries—none of which reduced sleep quality. But now with artificial lighting, we can stay up all night. Ever been to New York City's Time Square? Screens embedded into buildings makes it daylight all the time there. And bedrooms are like this, with constant exposure to screens through devices.

> **For better sleep, it's best to shut off all screens at least two hours prior to bed.**

We don't get enough natural light, which deters great health. Sunlight exposure during the day helps with restful sleep at night. Research shows that vitamin D is a missing component to quality sleep. Weight problems are also linked to vitamin D deficiency. Studies show that supplementation of 4,000 to 10,000 uL's of vitamin D can support more sleep.[50] Enough sunlight per day would be closer to 10,000 uL's of vitamin D.[51]

Screens pose another major threat to sleep. While there are benefits to blue light from screens, such as focus, there's tremendous research that proves blue light reduces the quality of sleep, quantity of sleep, and melatonin secretion.[52] For better sleep, it's best to shut off all screens at least two hours prior to bed.

Sleep Tight

In addition to the suggestions in this chapter, my best sleep advice is to practice body, soul, and spirit care. The body habits, as well as emotional fitness and spiritual disciplines, support healthy sleep.

Also, place boundaries around your bedtime. Figure out that perfect evening regimen that helps you to snooze blissfully through the night.

Don't let sleep rule you either. Not getting my sleep used to stress me out. At times I felt led to pray in the midnight hour. I wanted to be obedient to the Holy Spirit when prompted to pray. But I was a little mad at praying for the same old people with the same issues that I needed to intercede for them about in the late hours. I had to let go of my need for sleep in service to the Holy Spirit and others. Use wisdom and have grace with yourself and others in the matter. When you wake up in the early morning you may have need to pray too.

Sweet Dreams

Sleep is important, not only naturally but spiritually.

Dreams are a primary way Spirit speaks to people. I've had prophetic dreams since I was a child. Sometimes my sleep issues are a call to pray because insight from the Spirit needs to get to me via REM sleep.

There's a Biblical reference that God said, He'd pour out His Spirit on all people and we would have dreams (Joel 2:29). Check out fun reads like Jim Goll's *Dream Language* or Adam Thompson's *The Divinity Code to Understanding Your Dreams and Visions* to better interpret what God may be speaking to you.

And yes, sometimes dreams are because of an ice cream and pizza binge, but you'll look forward to going to sleep when you get to see a movie in your mind.

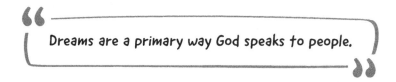

> Dreams are a primary way God speaks to people.

Be mindful of the physiological trigger of poor sleep going forward. Personally, it's my hardest habit to master, but we need to keep pressing forward in the pursuit of health. Are you with me?

Tips to Habitize Sleep

- Create a bedtime routine and stick to it most nights.
- Eat three to four hours before bedtime to support lower insulin and cortisol levels.

- Take time before bed to thank God for all He did in your day and is doing in your life. Gratitude generates better sleep vibes.

- Research natural supplementation to improve sleep quality if needed. A sleep oriented herbal tea with herbs like chamomile, valerian, skull-cap, kava kava, or uva ursi may help. Or try magnesium, tryptophan, ashwagandha, or melatonin supplements. Sleep medication is linked to premature death. [53] Given our goal is abundant life, sleep meds may be counterproductive.

- Try apps that stimulate REM brain waves. Brainwaves, Theta and Delta, can help to get us into deep sleep. Punch Delta or Theta sleep into YouTube for soothing sounds.

- Have a cut off time for electronic devices at least two hours before bed.

- Get the temperature right. The best temperature for sleep is 68 degrees or cooler.

- Do your best to drink water during the day and take your last pee right before you go to bed. Peeing in the middle of the night can be problematic to get back to sleep.

- Figure out ways to support your spouse's sleep including regular sexual relations, which releases oxytocin. Oxytocin reduces cortisol and stress.[54]

- If you didn't get the spiritual gift of sleep either, listen to Shawn Stevenson's enjoyable book *Sleep Smarter* on Audible for more tips.

REFLECT & SHARE

1. How would you rate the quality of your sleep?

_____

_____

_____

_____

_____

2. What time do you need to get to bed to ensure seven to eight hours of sleep?

_____

_____

_____

_____

_____

3. What types of bedtime boundaries do you need to put in place?

_____

_____

_____

_____

_____

CHAPTER 11

HABIT #5 EXERCISE
AM I INACTIVE?

Physiological Trigger – Inactivity

*Get fit and stay fit, not zero percent
body fat but enough to outrun a street cat.*

The first time I ran a 10k race I was about twelve years old. It went something like this.

"You want to come run a 10k for cancer with me in Philadelphia?" Aunt Lori asked over the phone.

"Yes, Aunt Lori, I can't wait!" I replied.

"Great, I'll pick you up Sunday at six o'clock in the morning. Be ready," she said and hung up.

Eager to hang out with my cool Aunt Lori, I didn't know what a 10k cancer run was, but it sounded good and noble, so why not? With no training and tight sneakers, it took me hours to run the 10k. I'll never forget the energy drain of the last mile. How I must've looked like such a goober, running with wild, large leg and arm movements in desperation, pleading for the finish line, rapidly panting until I got there.

I couldn't go to school the next day because the alarm went off and my arms, legs, and back refused to move. *Oh no, I'm paralyzed!* I thought. Panic set in. A scary moment as to be expected from a young person who piddled around from time to time with Mom's Jane Fonda workouts but never ran a 10k or a 1k anywhere.

I was so grateful when I realized I wasn't paralyzed. Nope, just young and dumb. My poor feet were smuggled into tight, new, black Nike sneakers in an attempt to make my big feet look smaller to peers. Blisters, black toe nails, and an aching body chased me for the rest of the week.

As a kid you don't think about weight or calories burned. I'd dance for hours in my bedroom because I loved to dance. It was easy to get lost in the joy of movement. Somewhere inside my head my desire to dance changed into a desire to lose weight. This switch made exercise a chore. It's like reading a book for homework. No one wants to do homework, but everyone wants to read what they want to read.

Children have boundless energy. As children we danced, jumped, swam, and annoyed adults to no end because adults can't keep up. Where did this energy go? What did you do as a kid for play? How can your kid play work for you in adulthood?

Inactivity Facts

1. A 2016 study of more than 1.44 million men and women showed that regular exercise decreased the risk of thirteen types of cancers, including liver, lung, breast, and colon cancers.[1]

2. Ages forty and up make up 50 percent of marathon finishers in the U.S. these days. In 1980, this figure was only 26 percent.[2]

3. Exercising for any amount of time reduces the premature death risk by 20 percent. Exercising thirty minutes most days reduces death by 31 percent. And exercising for ninety minutes most days reduces early death risk by 39 percent.[3,4]

4. Roughly 80 million Americans live a sedentary lifestyle.[5]

5. Any amount of strength training resulted in a lower body mass index and better eating, a 30 percent decrease in the risk of diabetes, and a 17 percent lower cardiovascular disease risk.[6]

6. People who do strength and cardio/aerobics at least 120 minutes per week lower their chance of diabetes by 65 percent.[7]

7. Ninety percent of people who have kept off thirty pounds or more do an hour of exercise most days.[8]

8. A study of women who walked each week had a 42 percent drop in breast cancer mortality risk.[9]

9. Disability risk is cut by 50 percent by walking.[10]

10. A high intensity interval workout for one minute can improve endurance and lower blood pressure.[11]

Do you wonder why someone hasn't invented the exercise-for-you robot yet in this technically advanced millennium? The odds of that happening are pretty low. If you want the benefits of exercise, you'll be the one who has to *do* the exercise.

Once you start, don't stop.

And once you start, don't stop.

The National Weight Control Registry showed that one hour of exercise most days was a causal factor to permanent weight release. [12]

If you've mastered this habit, well done! If not, we've got to get this habit down, albeit not at the expense of other body habits.

Nature's Remedy

Exercise is a miracle drug. And it's free. Like water, sleep, cleansing, and nutrition, activity is another natural remedy to a whole host of problems. With modern vehicles, we forget we have miracle wheels of our own,

We forget we have miracle wheels of our own, legs.

legs. One study of 80,000 females reduced their risks of cancer by 45 percent just by walking.[13]

The case for exercise is overwhelming. Exercise reduces the risk of more than thirteen types of cancer.[14] Exercise boosts mood and productivity and reduces anxiety and depression.[15] It reduces the effects and appearance of aging and extends life on average by four and a half years.[16,17] And exercise is so potent a medicine, it both prevents and reverses high blood pressure and diabetes.[18,19,20]

The best combo of exercise is a mix of cardio and strength training a couple times per week, which decreases the risk of diabetes by as much as 65 percent.[21] And any amount of strength training resulted in lower body mass index and better eating, a 30 percent decrease in diabetes risk, and a 17 percent lower cardiovascular disease risk.[22]

One study of mice that were near death divided the sick mice into two groups. One group exercised while sick and the other stayed sedentary. The mice who exercised three times per week regained strength and vitality. And they looked no different than the healthy mice despite their terminal illness.[23]

> **Unless you're LeBron James, you have no business spending all day exercising when there's not millions attached.**

Get Started

If you're an exerciser already, focus on other habits. But if it's arduous to think about moving off the couch in the evenings, don't worry about it. Studies show that diet alone can create powerful health outcomes. But those who exercise and don't change their diet won't get all the benefits.

When your energy shifts from mastering the body habits, you'll be compelled to move. It seems hard to get started, but most marathon runners start over the age of forty. Be the exception. Bryan Reese, at age forty-seven, broke his thirty-year sedentary lifestyle to complete three Ironmans, which involve a 2.4 mile swim, a 112 mile bicycle ride, and 26.2 mile marathon run.[24] Be inspired. It's better late than never.

The World Health Organization recommends we get 150 to 300 minutes of exercise per week or 30 to 60 minutes five days per week.[25] The key here is not to associate weight loss with

> " The primary excuse for not exercising is a lack of time. Don't buy this. "

workouts. I know, it's counterintuitive. But therein lies a big problem.

Shows, like the *Biggest Loser,* make us think exercise is the only way to lose weight. But the biggest losers worked out six to seven hours every day![26] Um, yeah. That's ridiculous. Unless you're LeBron James, you have no business spending all day exercising when there's not millions attached.

Ideally, we can dedicate one hour a day and combine it with some worship music or Bible study via an app because we know that exercise is mega-profitable, but not at the expense of godliness (1 Timothy 4:8). But all of the super fit people I know work out for two hours a day or do long workouts a couple times a week. And half of these people are in the fitness business—again a payment is attached.

Other research showed up to 450 minutes per week, or up to ninety minutes five days per week, was more beneficial.[27] I agree that some days I need more exercise and thrive on it. But this isn't always realistic or recommended in modern life, nor is it sustainable if you consider walking from the car to the front door a workout at the moment.

The primary excuse for not exercising is a lack of time.[28] Don't buy this. Chris walked every time he made a phone call. You can trade all the television time for sneakers, and you'll burn 120 calories more per day.[29]

Studies show a simple five-minute brisk walk once an hour can do the trick of reducing cravings and elevating mood.[30] One minute of ultra-intense exercise, like running upstairs a few times per week, delivered positive health improvements.[31]

For me, friends, sometimes I work out five minutes, and my mantra is something is better than nothing. On some days five minutes may be all you have. Just do your best and create the quantity that's realistic for you.

I also suggest finding activities you enjoy doing with loved ones. When you enjoy an activity, like basketball, tennis, or running, you're more likely to be consistent. This is especially true for female exercisers.[32] Workouts like pickleball are gaining traction for women because it's a sporty kind of fun.

Make it your mission to find something you love to do, such as dance, kickbox, or CrossFit. Try things until something jazzes you and do it often.

Move Motivation

Going forward, associate exercise with more short-term benefits to motivate yourself to do it. Short-term results are more motivating than longer term possible outcomes like weight loss.

First, mood. An immediate benefit is a happier mood for up to twenty four hours.[33] You may grunt the first ten minutes, but within twenty minutes of cardio exercise, significant physiological benefits occur and endorphins increase to buoy the worst of moods.[34]

Depressed adults who did forty-five minutes of cardio three times per week improved their mood more than Zoloft (an antidepressant).[35] Exercise combined with water and nutrition will make you feel like your younger self in no time.

Second, productivity. When you need to get things done, exercise is one way to do it. Exercise improves blood flow to the brain, so people feel more productive because they learn faster and have a better memory.[36] Studies show that people who strength train had a better ability to plan and organize.[37] It also wards off Alzheimer's. Exercise also helps you accomplish more tasks in a day. Those who exercise think better and have better memory retrieval.[38]

Third, reduced appetite for junk foods. Studies show that people eat better when they exercise because they don't crave as much junk food.[39] I find all these benefits for myself.

Besides reducing other negative health risks, exercise is one thing you can do to improve your body image, body mass index, self-esteem, and overall happiness.[40]

We're made to move.

When healthier, you'll want to move, walk, run, skip—okay skip is a stretch, but you get my point. It's normal to want to move. It's abnormal not to. I'll share with you why it's been difficult to want to exercise in Habit 6.

> " We're made to move.

Keep energy at the forefront. Focus on fitness itself. I mean, if you were chased right now, how far could you run? Get fit and stay fit, not zero percent body fat, but enough to outrun a street cat.

To get motivated, attach money to it. One study took money away from one group of participants (individually) each day they missed exercising. Money loss proved to be the best form of motivation compared with money gained.[41]

Put it into action, give your accountability partner 100 bucks for the month, and every time you miss working out, you lose three bucks while they keep it. That'll motivate you to hightail it outside. You can also try entering a competition. Nowadays there are apps that provide fitness challenges, or you can check out your workplace health incentive programs.

If you've failed at exercise attempts in the past, it's easy to think of excuses not to do it. You may think thoughts like I'm too busy, too big,

> " You're worth the try, try, try, try until you succeed strategy that's available by the grace of God.

too lazy, too scared, or too tired. You've probably taken a defibrillator to your dead exercise goal to revive it every January 1st, only to stop January 3rd. You're tired of making promises to yourself that you can't keep.

I get it.

But you know what, you're worth the try, try, try, try until you succeed strategy that's available by the grace of God. Start small but start. Go for consistency. Calendar activity five to six days per week. Work used to be physical; therefore, we had activity built into our daily lives. But if you're not a farmer working sun up to sun down physically, you've got to get moving.

Start slow. It doesn't make sense to start off too strong because it's unsustainable.

A man, about sixty years old, came into the gym. From his attire, it looked like he hadn't worked out since the '80s. He sported tube socks up to his knees, canary yellow short shorts, a sweat band around his head, and wristbands. Since the fashion police weren't around, he started the treadmill at about six miles per hour, and shortly after, he turned red, was fighting to breathe, and sweating bullets, not to the oldies.

Meanwhile, I was on the treadmill next to him, praying to God he wouldn't have a heart attack, *Oh God, please, please, please don't let him die right here!* Suddenly, he stopped running, grabbed his gym bag, and left. I saw him months later, which provided relief, but don't be like that guy scaring innocent bystanders into heart palpitations. Start slow. Walk before you run, because slow and steady wins the race.

Next is a list of creative ways to get moving. As you review the list, check for excitement in your heart. When you decide what you like, be consistent using the sticker strategy.

Fun Checklist

What types of activities below seem to generate natural interest? Check all that apply.

☐ Complete a 5k	☐ Get a dog and walk it three times a day	☐ Learn to rollerblade
☐ Adult night at the skating rink	☐ Row at your local row club	☐ Jog around a lake or park
☐ Walk whenever you talk on the phone in evenings	☐ Tennis with people from meetup.com	☐ Plan a paintball visit
☐ Hit balls at the driving range	☐ Try Zumba	☐ Play volleyball with a church group
☐ Join a church league basketball team	☐ Join a men's or women's soccer group	☐ Worship dance in your house
☐ Flag football	☐ Hike the closest trails	☐ Hit homeruns at the batting cage
☐ Mountain bike in the woods	☐ Indoor rock climbing	☐ Salsa dance lessons
☐ Attend a ballroom dance event	☐ Line or country dancing	☐ Join a running group
☐ Walk around the city with friends	☐ Ride a bike-a-thon	☐ Test out a kickboxing workout

The Sticker Strategy

In 2009, I finally got fed up with my yo-yo exercising. That's when you exercise for a day and then you're off the next year. I decided to do what Jerry Seinfeld did with writing. He focused on his writing consistency. Each day he wrote, he gave himself an X on a wall calendar where he could see it.[42]

I did the same thing, but with stickers. Positive reinforcement when I did exercise and indifference (not self-condemnation) when I didn't paved the way for more grace, healing, wholeness, and exercise consistency in my life.

Despite popular belief, you and I both know it takes a lot longer than twenty-one days to form the exercise habit. So, I used the sticker strategy for two years. And this year I'm celebrating ten years of working out three to six days per week for fifty weeks per year.

I also recommend you track for at least one full year and post in the *www.thechubbychurch.com* group when you've celebrated your first year.

Devices or apps for tracking are fine too, but old school, visible stickers are amazing. Yes, the smiley face ones, emoji's, heck, even stickers of ice cream or burgers. Get it done and post a sticker. Positive reinforcement works in pre-school through the lifespan to geriatric day care. Enjoy tracking, however you do it.

Be consistent. Whether you start with once a week or five days a week, be consistent. The sooner you start, the sooner the habit forms.

Also stay focused on body habits, especially nutrition, because you can't outrun a poor diet. And be mindful of not over-exercising because this could be a possible sign of an eating disorder called bulimia.

 Positive reinforcement works in pre-school through the lifespan to geriatric day care.

Bulimics may work out for many hours per day to burn off yesterday's binge eating episode. They do so to keep a normal weight. If you're prone to this, set a limit of ninety minutes on your exercise. I'll equip you with insight on compensatory eating behaviors in Book 2.

Jesus Walked

Walking is a hidden spiritual discipline that Christ demonstrated throughout the Scriptures. Jesus and the disciples didn't have the luxury of a car to ride around in or a desk job. They walked for miles per day. I know their movement strengthened them spiritually. Test it for yourself to see if exercise strengthens you spiritually.

Exercise is a spiritual discipline. It brings too much body, soul, and spirit health not to be.

People, like my friend Chris Natzke, leadership coach and author of *Black Belt Leadership*, did the *Camino de Santiago*. Also called *The Way of Saint James* because the path leads to a cathedral built in his honor. The Camino de Santiago is an early Christian pilgrimage in which Saint James traveled to preach the gospel in Spain.[43]

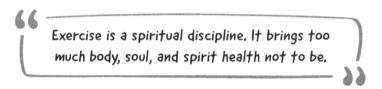

Exercise is a spiritual discipline. It brings too much body, soul, and spirit health not to be.

Over 100,000 people still do this spiritual path annually for the enlightenment it brings.[44] Most start at the French-Spanish border and travel parts or all of the inspirational 500 mile journey. People typically walk ten to thirty miles per day and fellowship with strangers on the common path of life.

I love to walk and run. But I use exercise to set my heart right for the day. A run outside with worship music on opens my heart for being more in the Spirit's flow the rest of the day. It doesn't replace quality time with the Lord, but it's a great combination. Not only is my heart in a more loving space, my prayer times are deeper. And my worship is stronger. Exercise connects us back to our healthiest identity of who we are.

Tips to Habitize Exercise

- Track progress using the sticker strategy, a device, or app to positively reinforce progress.
- Schedule your exercise on the calendar to increase your chance of getting it done.
- Combine prayer, worship music, and/or Scripture reading (apps) first thing in the morning.

- Join a gym with accountability. New fitness training centers are popping up everywhere, some require you to sign up for classes and pay a fee if you miss it. If there is no gym in your town, try apps like *StickK.com*.

- Start small, aim for five to ten minute walks, and each month increase that number.

- Unlink exercise from weight loss and link it to other immediate benefits, such as productivity, confidence, eating less junk, energy, or a happy mood.

- Routinize your exercise by making it a part of a daily routine. Don't think about it. Most of our delay is because we think ourselves out of doing it. Decide in the morning, jump out of bed, and get to it before you can talk yourself out of it.

- Find a fit friend to tag along with. We tend to become like the people we hang out with. You can join running groups, walking groups, or hiking clubs to meet fit people. Many faith focused fitness groups are on *meetup.com*.

- Make it competitive or join a fitness team. Research shows competition provides better results than social exercising.[45]

- Adopt the mantra "something is better than nothing" on days you don't want to do anything. Also pray. Plenty of times, I've asked the Holy Spirit to help me work out when motivation waned, and it works every time. Use exercise as a way to grow in the fruit of temperance.

- Enjoy your exercise. Stop forcing yourself to run if you hate it. It's harder to sustain exercise you don't enjoy. Be active. You don't have to burn a thousand calories. Just move. Hey, you can work out first then sit as your reward, fair?

REFLECT & SHARE

1. Which tip to habitize exercise do you want to try next?

_____

_____

_____

_____

_____

2. How long have you desired to make exercise a part of your daily routine?

_____

_____

_____

_____

3. How can you increase your activity within your lifestyle?

_____

_____

_____

_____

_____

CHAPTER 12

HABIT #6 BALANCE
AM I HORMONAL?

Physiological Trigger – Hormonal Imbalance

Insulin conserves our energy.
It says, "I've sat and I can't get up."

Gentlemen, please don't skip this habit assuming it doesn't pertain to you. Insulin, estrogen, cortisol, thyroid, testosterone—hormones affect us all. The fifty odd hormones that make up our endocrine system are major predictors of our vitality.

As we age these potent regulatory messengers send signals that change our energy, weight, and mood. Think about it, too much estrogen and a man will grow breasts. Too much testosterone and a woman will grow a beard.

Hormones are powerful.

Like a hurricane, when out of balance they swoop in and wipe out our efforts for better health. Hormonal imbalances are the strongest physiological triggers that directly impact emotional health, eating decisions, and weight.

> " *Hormonal imbalances are the strongest physiological triggers that directly impact emotional health, eating decisions, and weight.* "

Hormonal Imbalance Facts

1. Caffeine increases epinephrine, norepinephrine, and hormones that affect weight, cortisol, and insulin.[1]

2. In men, unforgiveness raised cortisol and aged them.[2]

3. Men experience 20 percent declines in testosterone each decade after the age of thirty-five.[3]

4. An estimated 52 percent of Americans have an underactive thyroid function.[4]

5. Women with hormonal imbalance consume 275 percent more refined sugar than women who are hormonally balanced.[5]

6. Cortisol, insulin, estrogen, testosterone, and the thyroid all affect body mass.[6]

7. Exercise increases testosterone for up to three hours after a workout.[7]

8. Alcohol has a direct negative impact on the liver, brain, hormones, and blood sugar. Eliminate or reduce alcohol consumption to balance cortisol, estrogen levels, and your risk of cancers.[8]

9. Sperm counts dropped in half between 1973 and 2011 in North America, Europe, Australia, and New Zealand.[9]

10. Experts estimate that 47 million Americans have metabolic syndrome, a symptom of hormonal imbalances.[10]

Endurance to exercise, energy to meal plan, or enthusiasm to take back our health from snaccidents is difficult with hormonal imbalance. Hormones decline as we age, but with the Standard American Diet, endocrine disruptor chemicals, and hormones in conventional animal foods, our hormones decline sooner.[11,12,13] Body fat needs vary for men and women, which tells us that sex hormones go into the process of storing body fat.[14]

More than 50 percent of women who reduced caloric intake and exercised over a two-month period couldn't reduce body fat due to hormonal imbalances.[15] Hormonal imbalance symptoms take many forms like unexplained weight gain or loss, excessive water retention, hair coarseness, dryness, or loss, sleep problems, fertility challenges, and more. Endocrine system problems coexist with most chronic diseases.

Hormones get out of balance for several reasons we've already discussed like consuming highly refined processed foods and beverages, dehydration, inadequate activity, micronutrient deficiency, poor sleep, endocrine disruptors, and environmental toxins.

Another contributor is the meat supply.

The Meat Supply

All animal foods have some level of hormones by nature. However, since 1950 the FDA has approved hormonal steroids in both natural and synthetic forms.[16] In 1993, Recombinant Bovine Growth Hormone (rBGH also labeled rBST) was introduced to get meat to market faster. It's reported that it's injected in about 80 percent of cattle.[17] I would suspect this percentage from any fast food joint, but in the grocery version the USDA reports less than 17 percent of cows are treated.[18]

The problem is these meat hormones affect our hormones. Conventional meat and dairy versus organic grass fed is one of the biggest disruptors in hormonal management. Vegans I've interviewed report that they feel hormonally balanced as a direct outcome of not eating animal foods.[19]

The milk from cows given rBGH are a risk factor for cancer tumor growth because these hormones increase Insulin-like Growth Factor (IGF-1), which is proven to increase the risks of prostate, breast, and colon cancers.[20,21]

Concerns, like sperm quality reduction, higher rates of prostate and breast cancer, and early onset puberty seem to be consequences of hormonally charged meat and dairy.[22,23,24] Our meat is also pumped with antibiotics, which goes back to Habit 1's gut issues, because they live in concentrated animal feeding operations that have abominable, inhumane practices.

Don't get me wrong. I love a good, well-done steak. God did, too! (Leviticus 1:1–17). But consider organic, grass fed. Grass fed has more nutrients and doesn't use hormones to beef it up.[25]

Let's do basic education on what hormonal imbalances cause problems.

> " Insulin's primary function is to get glucose into cells and store fat. "

Hormones to Balance

Insulin

Dr. Jason Fung, in his book *The Obesity Code: Unlocking the Secrets of Weight Loss,* called out insulin resistance as the reason for obesity. Fung says, "Obesity is a hormonal dysregulation of fat accumulation."[26]

He refers to a weight set point like a thermostat stuck on a temperature. Our weight set point is very difficult to turn down because of insulin resistance. Insulin's primary function is to get glucose into cells and store fat.

Insulin is often described as a key to unlock cells so that glucose (blood sugar) can get into the cell. When insulin resistance occurs, insulin is unable to unlock cells for the group of glucose molecules to go inside. Insulin may be able to let one or two of them in the cell door, but the rest hang out on the front lawn.

And if glucose can't get into liver or muscle cells to be utilized for fuel, insulin sends the rowdy glucose molecules into neighboring fat cells. Kind of like if you couldn't get into your house because you were locked out, you'd go to your neighbor's house. Glucose that can't get in, goes to fat cells to hang out there instead.

The pancreas pumps insulin to handle the excess glucose in the system, becoming impaired. Insulin signals the body to eat more to support its glucose fat storage efforts. This translates into body mass growth and energy conservation.

It's an explanation for those worn butt prints on the sofa. Insulin conserves our energy. It's says, "I've sat, and I can't get up."[27] Hence, when insulin resistance occurs, it's very difficult to want to do much. A spiritual word for this is laziness. Insulin resistance promotes weight gain and lethargy. We want insulin sensitivity, not resistance. Insulin sensitivity is when cells welcome insulin to unlock their door so more glucose can get in.

High blood sugar is one indicator of insulin resistance. In a fasting blood glucose test, pre-diabetic levels that range between 100 mg/dl and 125 mg/dl are usually insulin resistant. Diabetics' blood fasting glucose is 126 mg/dl or higher.[28]

When insulin levels are high, it's almost impossible to release weight. We can gather this from research that shows insulin treatment for diabetes causes weight gain.[29] One study showed as much as nineteen pounds gained within six months.[30] And if you take insulin, you've probably seen this for yourself. Insulin as a correction may not be the best solution, especially since obesity and weight is a precursor to diabetes.

You're aware that processed foods, snacks, candies, and soda are rough for blood sugar, but they also alter hormones, all hormones. Dr. Fung says, "Refined carbohydrates, such as white sugar and white flour, cause the greatest increase in insulin levels."[31] When one hormone is out of balance it ricochets on the others too.

Some people are carbophobes (deathly afraid of carbohydrates in any form), but the type of carbohydrate makes a radical difference in fat storage. You can eat as many green beans as you want and as long as they're not smothered in gooey cheese you won't gain weight, but you'll likely release weight and certainly improve your health.

But those sugary corn muffins, expect weight gain a few hours after consumption. Let me tell you, I'm a huge fan of corn bread so I know this from personal experience. Furthermore, every time we eat, we increase insulin levels. But, those of us overweight or obese increase insulin twice as much when we eat compared with healthy weight eaters.[32]

Said another way, one of Fung's forerunners, Gary Taubes, author of *Why We Get Fat: And What To Do about It*, likens fat tissue growth to growing height. Like growth hormones are programmed to help us reach a certain height, insulin and other hormones drive us to store fat.[33]

> " Those of us overweight or obese increase insulin twice as much when we eat compared with healthy weight eaters. "

Overeating (gaining caloric energy) and lethargy (conserving caloric energy) is caused by our hormonal drive to store fat. A long-distance runner is driven to burn the energy of stored fat, whereas others through diet are driven to create fat instead. Taubes proves that it's the fat processing mechanisms from the dietary intake of chemicals and refined edible delights, especially high fructose corn syrup (HFCS), that throws our fat storage processing into overdrive.[34]

All fructose must be converted into glucose in the liver. Excess is converted to fat.[35] HFCS is considered the easiest to convert into fat as well because unlike fruit fructose, it has no binding agent to slow down metabolism.

When you drink soda with HFCS you speed up the metabolic process of fructose to fat, a major culprit of fatty liver disease.[36,37] Fructose consumption used to be half a pound per year in our diets from fruit, which is positive, but in recent years we're eating over sixty pounds of fructose per person from processed foods and drinks, which is negative.[38]

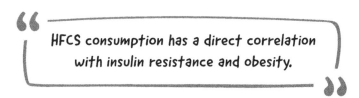

> " HFCS consumption has a direct correlation with insulin resistance and obesity. "

HFCS consumption has a direct correlation with insulin resistance and obesity.[39] Unless we're in an end times apocalypse and food is scarce (which in that case grab a box of Twinkies® and run for the hills), please don't eat or drink it.

Besides increasing fiber intake (see Habit 2), Dr. Fung recommends intermittent fasting—the practice of giving your blood fasting insulin and glucose levels time to heal.[40]

To balance her hormones at sixty, Ann started intermittent fasting in July. By February of the next year, she had released eighteen pounds. Two nights a week, she stopped eating at seven o'clock and wouldn't eat again until eleven o'clock in the morning. This gave her hormones sixteen hours to get their balancing act together. She also overcame her processed food and sugar addiction to reduce hormonal effects.

Intermittent fasting is a fancy term for what used to be normal. In 1977, we ate three meals a day. Then meals were four and a half hours apart. Now we eat five to six times per day, with three and a half hours between meals or less.[41] Because we eat all day and night, insulin is always elevated. This makes our weight set point stay set on high.

Similar to a restaurant that gives patrons the opportunity to eat during operating hours, intermittent fasting has open feeding hours. When the feeding hours are over, the kitchen's closed.

This long period of fourteen to eighteen hours without food at night helps to heal elevated insulin levels. Although tasty, snacks aren't necessary. They're usually highly processed snaccidents waiting to happen anyway. Perhaps we balance by eating enough of the right stuff at meals to sustain not eating processed snacks between meals.

In the chart below ketones represent fat burn, and glucose represents sugar burn. The arrows represent meal times.

Although tasty, snacks aren't necessary. They're usually highly processed snaccidents waiting to happen anyway.

M.P. Mattson et al. / Ageing Research Reviews 39 (2017) 46–58

Figure 12.1 Fasting Glucose and Ketones[42]

In Chapter 17 we'll address the dieter's mindset so ideas like intermittent fasting don't become another fad diet. If you feel Spirit led to adopt this practice, try it once a week to start. An extreme approach usually causes weight gain recidivism. We'll cover more on fasting and food addiction in Book 2.

Insulin and cortisol are a dynamic duo when it comes to hormonal balance. When insulin's up, cortisol is also.

Cortisol

High cortisol increases insulin because it governs blood sugar.[43] It's also responsible for immune function and blood pressure.[44] We covered cortisol in Habit 4, but along with insomnia, other symptoms of high cortisol include a racing mind, strong task orientation, cravings for sugar after meals, the inability to go without food for four to six hours, over thirty-five inches around belly, edema, puffy face, bone loss, high blood sugar, high blood pressure, irregular cycles, or memory lapses.[45]

If you've wondered about belly fat, elevated cortisol is the culprit for missing buttons on pants. There's four times more cortisol receptors in the belly than elsewhere in the body.[46] Cortisol studies prove body mass index increases with higher levels of cortisol.[47] Those with high cortisol usually have high blood pressure and high glucose, since cortisol's job is to increase glucose and blood pressure.

To balance cortisol, practices of sleep and stress reduction work best. Remember from Habit 4, cortisol increases as much as 100 percent after one night of poor sleep.[48] So keep boundaries on bedtime.

Stress can be any sense of threat we feel. Gary Taubes said, "[Cortisol] may explain why some people get fatter when they get stressed, anxious, or depressed and eat more, and some people do the opposite."[49]

I call stressful event weight gain a *circumstantial trigger*. When we're going through a stressful event like divorce, a loved one dying, or a large financial expense, we experience weight gain for a period of time. Once the stressful circumstance is over, weight goes back to normal. This is the case with cortisol levels and stress.

In regard to stress hormones, Dr. Fung said, "Stress contains neither calories nor carbohydrates but can still lead to obesity." Do what you've got to do. Reduce commitments, manage a budget, work your life more

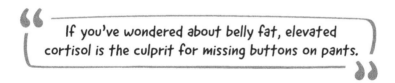

If you've wondered about belly fat, elevated cortisol is the culprit for missing buttons on pants.

through a calendar, and relieve stress. After all, that bumper sticker said, "You're too blessed to be stressed."

One outcome of elevated cortisol over time is adrenal fatigue. Adrenal fatigue speaks to chronically high cortisol and other stress hormones in the adrenals like adrenaline that make you feel exhausted, depressed, and anxious.[50]

It's a sign that the stores of stress hormones are depleted. Adrenal fatigue thwarts health efforts. One physical sign of adrenal fatigue is a darker indent around your eye sockets that seem to be sinking in. Reduce your stress to protect them from burn out or rebuild them if they already are.[51]

Thyroid

The thyroid is in the throat area near the larynx. Thyroid

> " Take your temperature each day for a week, and if it's under 97.8 degrees most days, you likely have low thyroid function. "

hormone is produced at the direction of the hypothalamus (the hormone divisional leader under the brain's leadership) and made by the pituitary gland, but also converted to active use in the gut, liver, and tissues.[52]

The thyroid is responsible for utilizing caloric energy in all cells and heartbeat regulation, affecting metabolism, weight, and mood.[53] Symptoms of a low thyroid are thinning outer eyebrows, hoarse voice, puffy face, fatigue, dry skin, weakness, often feeling cold, sleep problems, impaired memory, or slow speech.[54]

Nutritional deficiencies of iodine, tyrosine, zinc, selenium, vitamins A, C, D, B2, B3, B12, and healthy fats contribute to a slow thyroid because they aid in its function.[55,56] Take your temperature each day for a week, if it's under 97.8 degrees most days, you likely have low thyroid function.[57]

Have your doctor check for TSH, thyroid stimulating hormone. The higher the TSH the slower the thyroid function. A TSH level toward the middle or lower end of the range may alleviate symptoms.[58] The standard TSH normal in medical practice is below what current research shows is most effective for thyroid function, which is why many go undiagnosed.[59,60] You can also check T3 (active thyroid hormone) and T4 (thyroid hormone in storage which converts to T3 when needed).

Studies show that a higher TSH is associated with obesity, but researchers haven't found a causal reason why.[61] Some who take medication for thyroid don't see much of an effect on weight—probably because it wasn't causal to their weight symptom.[62]

Low thyroid influences weight, but the American Thyroid Association states that weight release is only effective for about 10 percent of weight gained pre-treatment.[63] This is why managing overall hormonal balance is a more effective strategy for weight and eating freedom. If weight releases with thyroid support medications, then the thyroid was likely the causal problem. If not, it's probably another condition.

Anthony William, author of *Thyroid Healing,* attributes thyroid symptoms to a low-grade Epstein Barr Virus (EBV) in the liver not being properly treated.[64] He suggests that the sixty variations of EPV that affect an estimated 225 million Americans are causal to mystery illnesses like fibromyalgia, chronic fatigue syndrome, and hypothyroidism.[65]

> " Thyroid health affects a gang of reproductive
> health complications in women, such as
> miscarriages, infertility, and still births. "

He attests that an autoimmune response in the thyroid, called Hashimoto's disease, may be your immune system fighting off an undiagnosed variation of EBV.[66] Ask your doctor to check thyroid antibodies and consider Anthony William's recommendations on healing naturally.

Another worthy mention is my shero, Dana Trentini. Dana's an award-winning, hypothyroid health activist who miscarried her baby because of what doctors didn't know about thyroid health.

She found in her research that the American Thyroid Association warns about pregnancy complications because of low thyroid.[67] She also found thyroid health affects a gang of reproductive health complications in women, such as miscarriages, infertility, and still births.[68]

She wrote, "Research reveals hypothyroidism is linked to heart disease, diabetes, Alzheimer's, cancer, issues with the liver, kidneys, gall bladder, mental health, pregnancy complications, and more."[69]

Thyroid medication shouldn't be looked at as a weight loss miracle solution. But thyroid support may be necessary in your pursuit of health. There are natural ways to increase thyroid function and hormone—like kelp granules sprinkled on food which provides iodine or iodine supplementation.

Iodine is necessary for optimal thyroid function and works to increase T4 which converts to T3. Fluoride interferes with thyroid hormone, and it's in our toothpaste and tap water. Use a non-fluoridated toothpaste and filtered water to support these efforts.[70]

Testosterone

> " If you feel like nothing excites or interests you, talk to your doctor about low-T. "

Testosterone has many functions in the body including libido, muscle development, strength, stamina, and energy.[71] Low testosterone (low-T) symptoms are less motivation, low energy, low libido, anxiety, irritability, low stamina, weak muscles, and poor muscle growth.[72]

I figured out I had low-T when I felt blah. I traveled a great deal for work at the time, which taxed my body. If you feel like nothing excites or interests you, talk to your doctor about low-T because low-T levels may increase the risk for diabetes as well.

In one study of 300 men, 40 percent had diabetes and low-T.[73] Of those men, 25 percent weren't obese. Low-T is a factor of sub-optimal health. Low-T is also associated with a high body mass index, diabetes and insulin resistance.[74]

Check your testosterone with blood work. For women, Dr. Sara Gottfried recommends optimal blood testosterone levels to be between 75–130 uL.[75] When I had the case of the blahs, mine was at 4 uL. For men, Dr. Anna Cabeca, recommends testosterone ranges between 300–1000 uL, with optimal levels between 600–800 uL.[76]

Andropause, the male version of menopause, is when testosterone levels decline in males. It starts at age thirty-five and causes testosterone levels to drop approximately 20 percent in each of the following decades.[77] Menopause starts on average at age fifty-one. Women may see drops in all sex hormone levels.[78]

After you get your blood work, don't be surprised if yours is low. Dr. Andre Harris, OBGYN, talked about his intimacy issues with his wife as a result of testosterone imbalance in his humorous TED talk. Low-T affected their marital happiness and libido, especially for his wife. For him, it affected his weight. He felt "fat, flabby, and fatigued."[79]

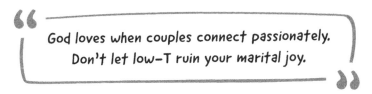

> God loves when couples connect passionately. Don't let low-T ruin your marital joy.

He decided to utilize testosterone pellets, rice-sized bio-identical hormones implanted under the skin to boost levels. It worked. He and his wife eliminated marital unhappiness and poor libido. In his words, "It was on and 'poppin'" in the bedroom. God loves when couples connect passionately. Don't let low-T ruin your marital joy.

Dr. Harris also had energy to exercise before or after the work day, which affected his weight. Synthetic testosterone hormones have negative effects. But bio-identical hormone treatments are a natural way to go if other (less pricey) solutions don't work.

Overall, if you find yourself weepy or watching the soap operas, you probably could use a bit more testosterone support. However, some older men I've talked to like their new found sensitive side and really enjoy *The Young and the Restless*, which brings me to our last hormone review.

Estrogen

Estrogen supports healthy bones, joints, and overall "juiciness" in the body as Dr. Sara Gottfried puts it in her comprehensive fabulous book, *The Hormone Cure*, geared toward women. Estrogen has a role in libido, body mass, and energy.[80] It's estimated that half of women over thirty-five are estrogen dominant, as well as anyone with a stubborn midsection.[81]

We want the optimal ranges of estrogen to be not too high and not too low. Estrogen has a direct effect on insulin resistance; therefore, it's a leading factor in body fat regulation.[82,83] Estrogen dominance can create health risk factors, including cancer, stroke, and thyroid dysfunction.[84]

By nature, fat cells produce estrogen. Obese men and women are typically estrogen dominant.[85] Dr. Anna Cabeca said, "The average sixty-year-old man has more circulating estrogen in his blood than the average sixty-year-old woman."[86] See, I wasn't kidding about the interest in soap operas in older men.

Estrogen dominance symptoms in women range from bloating, low libido, anxiety attacks, weight gain, insomnia, and memory lapses, to fuller breasts.[87] For men, signs are infertility, erectile dysfunction, and gynecomastia—the technical term for man boobs.[88] Estrogen can block thyroid function.[89]

> "Low estrogen is also pretty tough on couples in the love department."

Low estrogen symptoms, such as irritability, joint aches, dryness, and low libido, affect men and women.[90,91] Men may have erectile dysfunction.[92] And women may have vaginal dryness. Low estrogen is also pretty tough on couples in the love department.

Another problem with low estrogen is that it stimulates binge eating.[93] Estrogen balance keeps leptin (appetite control) in check, whereas estrogen deficiency pokes leptin to request food.[94]

> "Low estrogen stimulates binge eating."

In a study of rats who had their ovaries removed, the rats gained weight and only moved to get food, despite controls to stop overeating.[95] Ovaries are where estrogen is made in women. Although fed a normal amount of food, they gained weight. Once they were given estrogen all returned to normal, including their appetites and desire to move.

Similar to insulin, estrogen has a powerful effect on weight and eating behaviors. As Taubes quotes the researcher, "An animal doesn't get fat because it overeats, it overeats because it's getting fat."[96]

This is the power of our hormones.

And my lady friends, this explains why hormonal weeks are rough for binge eating desires because estrogen levels drop. See, overeating isn't because we're gluttons per say (we'll save the gluttony conversation for Book 2), but it's mostly a biological response.

You'll want to get your levels checked. Mayo Clinic suggests normal estrogen (as estradiol serum) ranges in women to be 13–350 pg/mL (postmenopausal about 40 pg/mL) and men between 10–40 pg/mL.[97] Dr. Sara Gottfried suggests women be in the top half of the range and postmenopausal women at 50 pg/mL for bone health.[98]

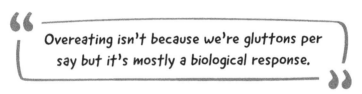

> Overeating isn't because we're gluttons per say but it's mostly a biological response.

Estrogenic foods may need to be eliminated. Nuances to estrogen balance are dairy and meat products. Dr. Josh Axe said, "The average U.S. citizen consumed 647 pounds of dairy. And anywhere from 60 to 80 percent of estrogens in the typical Western diet comes from milk and other dairy products. This is linked to a higher rate of testicular and prostate cancers."[99]

Soy can be a problem for estrogen and thyroid hormones, but the research is varied. Habit 2 facts note U.S. soy has genetically modified organisms (GMOs). Corn and wheat are also grown with GMOs.

Animal studies confirm that GMOs create tumors, cancers, and a host of other issues.[100,101] It's best to choose fermented non-GMO soy and organic non-GMO corn and wheat.

Keep Habit 2 in mind as BPA, dioxides, pesticides, phthalates, nonstick cookware, flame resistant chemicals, and so many more environmental chemicals mimic estrogen and attach to estrogen receptors creating toxic, bad girl strands of estrogen hormones called xenoestrogens.[102] These strands prevent real estrogen from working properly. Estrogen is especially sensitive to BPA.[103,104] Fiber intake helps keep your system clean from these toxins.

Supplements like Diindolylmethane (DIM), a phytonutrient derived from cruciferous vegetables, like cabbage and broccoli, are supportive in helping estrogens convert to testosterone and metabolize estrogen.[105]

Maca powder, put into smoothies, is effective for estrogen, thyroid, and testosterone imbalance symptom alleviation. It's also in the same vegetable family of cruciferous vegetables, like DIM, but it is grown in South America. Maca has proven results in reducing hormonal challenges like erectile dysfunction, infertility, muscle endurance, balancing estrogen, increasing muscle strength, and boosting libido.[106,107]

Consider natural remedies for the hormonal symptoms you have first. Powerful hormonal balancers, like DIM, maca powder, black cohosh, red ginseng, ashwagandha, holy basil, and rhodiola have proven results.

After you get blood work, research natural solutions to figure out which may work best for you. Synthetic hormone medications are extremely risky for sex hormones like estrogen and testosterone, do your homework first if they're prescribed.

Habitize Body Stewardship to Balance

Good news, you've learned the habits that best support hormonal balance, which is why I saved this habit for last. Keep things simple. Habitize Body Stewardship. Let's recap.

- Habit 1: **Nutrient Loading** supports hormonal balance because you get the building blocks hormones need. Vitamins, minerals, amino acids, and fatty acids all support hormonal function. Gut health is extremely important to proper nutrient absorption and hormone manufacturing.

- Habit 2: **Cleanse.** Hormones are converted in the liver. A clogged liver will affect hormone metabolism. A clean system helps to reduce xenoestrogens that create estrogen problems in men, women, and children.

- Habit 3: **Hydrate.** Hormones are messengers. To get the message to where it needs to go, they're transported. This happens through blood plasma, which is 90 percent water. Also, hormone molecules have a lifecycle. Water is vital to flush impaired molecules out of the system.

- Habit 4: **Sleep** is powerful to balance hormones, and you'll feel the effects the same day.

- Habit 5: **Exercise** is extra potent for all hormones, but specific types of exercise may benefit specific hormones. For example, walking, tai chi, and stretching help thyroid function and reduce cortisol.[108] To unleash more testosterone, reduce insulin, and balance estrogen, consider tough workouts like high intensity interval training (HIIT) and weight training.[109] A mix may be best because cortisol increases with exercise. Per Habit 5, frequency produces the most balanced results.

- Habit 6: **Balance.** Habitize body habits 1, 2, 3, 4, and 5, and the following tips.

The discussed hormones aren't the only ones to balance, but they're a great start. Focus on the fundamentals and allow your health to transform.

Tips to Habitize Hormonal Balance

- Habitize Body Stewardship. Each of the body habits are vital to hormonal balance. Eat green vegetables daily, cleanse your organs, drink plenty of water, prioritize sleep, and exercise for your hormones to naturally balance.

- Take time to rest. Take a day to completely rest once a week to restore your spirit and soul. A Sabbath has healing blessings (Isaiah 58:8,13).

- Get your hormonal blood work done. Ask for free and blood testosterone, full thyroid panel, estrogen, and a full metabolic panel. It's best to use a bio-identical hormone specialist or functional medicine physician.

- Take at least five minutes a day to destress. Read, walk, unplug, stretch, or share your heart with someone.

- Monitor your hormonal cycles by tracking moods on the calendar.

- Try alternative therapies. Alternative therapies such as acupuncture, massage, and contemplative prayer meditation are effective at balancing hormones.

- Reduce or eliminate caffeine consumption.

- Increase protein consumption (plant-based ideal) to 20 to 30 grams per meal.[110]

- Ladies check out *The Hormone Cure* by Dr. Sara Gottfried to keep learning. Gentlemen, consider sites like Dr. Jade Teta's Metabolic effect at *metaboliceffect.com* or Dr. Anna Cabeca at *drannacabeca.com.*

- *Bonus Tip:* To the ladies that suffer with premenstrual syndrome (PMS), Lorraine Pintus, co-author of *Intimate Issues*, has an excellent, Christ-centered book around cultivating healthy attitudes around hormones, appropriately called *Jump off the Hormone Swing.* An estimated 90 percent of women experience PMS and 5 percent suffer debilitating symptoms.[111] Please consider if you want deeper healing on the matter.

REFLECT & SHARE

1. How well do you manage your hormones?

_____

_____

_____

_____

_____

2. Do you notice when your hormonal balance is off?

_____

_____

_____

_____

_____

3. What tip(s) can you try to balance?

_____

_____

_____

_____

_____

CHAPTER 13

PRIORITIZE BODY CARE

The best caregivers honor their body, soul, and spirit.

Just like you'd prioritize an appointment with your boss at work, do the same with your body care.

Our mission can be cut short because we don't prioritize body stewardship. Our health is a priority. Otherwise we'll prioritize it for the wrong reasons.

I'll repeat again, if we don't make self-care a priority, we'll be in a position where someone will need to care for us. Someone like a nurse, spouse, or an adult child. Crisis lurks at the door for body neglectors.

You'll find it's true, that when you honor your body, it will honor you in return. You'll have more energy to serve others well. To love others as yourself.

> " *Crisis lurks at the door for body neglectors.* "

Nadine Roberts-Cornish, author of *Tears in My Gumbo: The Caregiver's Recipe for Resilience* said, "Love is the secret sauce in all the recipes of caregiving and is the healing source for our lives, for our world."[1]

Nadine understands how important it is for the caregiver to take care of others by making sure that we put our masks on first, as a flight attendant instructs. There are others in your life that you care for, give them your best. We're all caregivers to some degree, even if you only care for a plant.

The best caregivers honor their body, soul, and spirit.

Jesus took time to nurture Himself. He retreated into the wilderness or took walks alone to refresh. He served all of mankind.

The more we serve, the more critical it is to have adequate body, soul, and spirit care. Leaders know this. Many successful people nail these body habits. Body, soul, and spirit habits are critical for great success.

Nadine said to, above all, be driven by love. The love of God compels us to honor our temple, to refresh ourselves, and to care for others from His heart of love. Body habits support those efforts.

Chances are we'll need a caregiver at some point in our lives. Delay that point as long as you can. You have a destiny to attain. You have a purpose to fulfill. You have a calling in your life. And you have people that love you and need your love to get them through life!

I wouldn't be as soul happy and healthy as I am without the love of my grandparents. One of the benefits of my mom having me at nineteen years old was being raised with five grandparents alive most of my life. My grandparents are my heart. Their wisdom and love nurtured calm in my life of chaos.

> " The more we serve, the more critical it is to have adequate body, soul, and spirit care. "

You are important. You matter! And it's my honor to serve you with these habits.

Each body habit supports one another. Each one has a dramatic impact on your health, weight, eating, and emotions.

Consider making them easy:

- You're already eating – add green vegetables.
- You're already bathing – just clean your insides (not with soap).
- You're already drinking – make it mostly water.

- You're already going to bed – make your bedroom an oasis.
- You're already hormonal – be intentional.

Seek progress, not perfection. When these habits become who we are, body care is easy.

Think of it this way, if Dwayne Johnson (The Rock), jumped inside of your body in a case of the body snatchers, do you think you'd be fit fairly quickly? Yes, indeed. He'd jump inside your body, run to the nearest gym, and start lifting weights!

After that he'd bake some fish and broccoli. Dwayne Johnson's identity drives him to be fit and eat well.[2] (But, technically, like Hercules, Dwayne Johnson is buff obese, just saying.) As you work on these habits, consider who you are. You are healthy.

To make it easier to adopt these habits, some people love an acronym for memory's sake. I've changed a few words to make a good acronym. Cheers to a win-win for both of us.

THE BODY H.A.B.I.T.S.

H: Hydrate
A: Activity (Exercise)
B: Balance (Hormones)
I: NutrIent Load
T: DeTox (Cleanse)
S: Sleep

Nice, huh? Take a few moments to memorize H.A.B.I.T.S.

Congratulations for reading to this point. You're serious about taking back your health, and it shows. Every page turned is a victory.

I urge you to consider joining us in the *www.thechubbychurch.com* to work on these habits with others. You'll get access to resources, as well as support to cheer on your transformation.

This journey takes time.

Every time you do something that honors your body, soul, and spirit, you're making progress in the right direction. Celebrate as you go, not with cake, but with a song and dance.

Every page turned is a victory.

Get great at managing your life. Prioritize body care. We're not done, but you have the basics for what to focus on daily. Keep reading. Get your freedom from this book. And get your victory in Book 2.

REFLECT & SHARE

1. How will you improve taking care of your temple?

_____

_____

_____

_____

2. Will you break the chain of body neglect in your life once and for all? How so?

_____

_____

_____

_____

_____

SOUL

CHAPTER 14

GRUBBOLOGY
SAY HELLO TO YOUR INNER GLUTTON

My Inner Glutton made me do it.

Welcome to Soul. Over the next several chapters we'll look at soul psychological aspects of the weight and eating equation. Because in regard to your relationship with food, you may have wondered, *Have I been crazy all this time and didn't know it?!* Don't worry, my friend, you're not crazy. For the purposes of this book, we'll assume you're relatively normal. But, the insanity inside of us is crazy.

Let's look at that sense of craziness this way: you have three parts within that keep the drama of weight and eating alive, and two of them are two sides of the same coin.

They are the:

Inner Glutton ⎫
   Diet Nut ⎬ Both Make Up the Bound Self
  Whole Self

Like a husband and wife are two people, but one unit, so is your Inner Glutton and Diet Nut. They're married—only it doesn't feel like holy matrimony, more like *Dr. Jekyll and Mr. Hyde.* They're part of the soul bound in fear, resistance, identity crisis, and the past. They operate distinctly. I'll explain both as we set up context for these psychological factors of weight and eating, Grubbology and her sister 'ology—Chubbology.

Let's start with your Inner Glutton.

Meet Your Inner Glutton

You know there's an Inner Glutton in you, but you may not have formally met. Allow me to introduce you. And, yes, I get you prefer to say goodbye, not hello, but to break free of weight and eating bondage, we'll need to get to know your Inner Glutton very intimately. Without conscious awareness, lasting change doesn't happen.

The Inner Glutton is the part of you overeating and engaging in other unwanted behaviors to sabotage health and weight. Most humans have one to some degree.

But our Inner Glutton may not show up as food choices for everyone. In our case, our Inner Glutton wants delicious food and finds herself in detention, written up for a case of food trouble. Without wisdom in the moment, she sabotages your healthy efforts. It's a story that goes just like my cookie story, only with your own version of cookie. The Inner Glutton is the part of us acting out of our hurting soul to meet internal unmet needs.

> **The Inner Glutton is the part of us acting out of our hurting soul to meet internal unmet needs.**

Our Inner Glutton sabotages in four distinct ways, he or she:

1. Eats too much. [An episode or binge is eating a large caloric volume within a two-hour time frame.]

2. Eats the wrong stuff. [Chooses food or drinks that cause problems mentally, physically, emotionally, spiritually, or otherwise.]

3. Avoids the right stuff. [Chooses to avoid food or drinks able to help solve problems mentally, physically, emotionally, spiritually, or otherwise.]

4. Neglects body stewardship.

Our weight and eating struggles exhaust our strength of will from this war within. Almost without any effort, we end up in a place of hopeless despair.

We resolve in our hearts:

"I'll always be this way."

"I must be made to be overweight."

"I'll never win so why try?"

"My whole family is like this, I don't stand a chance."

We then proceed to eat whatever, whenever.

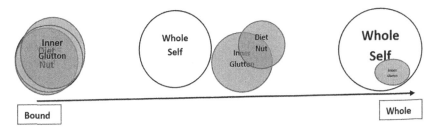

Figure 14.1 Process of Bound to Whole Self

In these cases, you and your Inner Glutton haven't begun the process of separation to integration. For some of us, the Inner Glutton is our identity. Like a Siamese twin, the lines are blurred between who our Inner Glutton is and who our whole self is.

We *are* the weight and eating struggle.

We really don't know who we are without excess fat, food crazies, binges, or dieting distractions. Consequently, we're unable to affect lasting change if our whole self isn't identifiable. Part of the vision work in The Call to Weight & Eating Freedom Action Plan was to align our hearts with our whole self.

> We really don't know who we are without excess fat, food crazies, binges, or dieting distractions.

It's also possible for the Inner Glutton to completely change faces and turn into a Diet Nut to attempt to control the out-of-control Inner Glutton side. All this mischievousness drives your whole self bonkers. You then doubt your ability to get healthy, stay healthy, and be healthy for life. And guys bear with me as I use the she pronoun to emphasize these distinctions.

Diet Nut – The Inner Glutton's Alter Ego

Meet Diet Nut. Your Inner Glutton does the sabotaging, and your Diet Nut devises diet plans to clean up the damage. Your Inner Glutton will eat all she wants on the weekends. Then Sunday night, Diet Nut gets fed up and kicks Inner Glutton back into shape on Monday, of course, with a strict, diet fix.

> Your Inner Glutton is childlike in nature, a rebel type, whereas your Diet Nut is a strict parent, a Pharisee type.

Your Inner Glutton is childlike in nature, a rebel type, whereas your Diet Nut is a strict parent, a Pharisee type. Your Inner Glutton engages in her antics and like a child says, "I'll eat whatever I want, when I want, and however much I want!" Then heads to the kitchen to bake brownies.

Diet Nut gets frustrated and says, "Why did you eat all those brownies? I can't stand you! It's all chicken and broccoli for you after this, missy!" As Diet Nut proceeds to research the latest get-skinny-quick plan.

Hence, the war within continues.

Understand this flipside of the coin because it's an all or nothing game—black or white, either all out-of-control [Inner Glutton] or all in-control [Diet Nut]. No grace. No balance. No love.

Our Diet Nut is the part of us that:

1. Devises diet plans. [Restricts eating, eats perfectly, and works out to death.]
2. Criticizes body parts, body shape, and size.
3. Distracts us from dealing with soul wounds.
4. Controls an out-of-control identity crisis.

Your Whole Self – A Health Warrior

Your whole self supersedes your Inner Glutton and Diet Nut. It's the part of you seeking freedom for lasting change, permanent weight release, and energy to do good for the kingdom's sake.

It's the part reading this book or committed to the Whole & Free Health course. It's the part that operates out of God's love and is highly connected with God's Spirit. It's your authentic identity. The real you. Whole Self emerges when your sense of identity of feeling broken or bound is cleared up. Because the truth of your identity is you're not broken or bound.

And my, oh my, is it tough to hear your true voice. When she's screaming her truth, we order a big ol' burrito to tune her out. We miss her heart's need and live in this unrelenting cycle of shame and guilt.

> **Because the truth of your identity is you're not broken or bound.**

Grubbology
(noun) Grub-ba-lo-gy
the made up psychological study of why we overeat

151

At this point, you're probably wondering how to get away from your Inner Glutton. But before you chase her down the street with a machete, screaming, "Stop sabotaging me, you demon child!" – know your Inner Glutton isn't to be shamed.

She's to be observed.

After all, you've shamed her enough all these years, and it doesn't create a healthier body or a happier you. She wants you to pay attention. She wants you to see her asking for your help to fulfill a need.

Your Inner Glutton is a wise teacher.

She's teaching you about your need be it spiritual, relational, emotional, physical, mental, and even financial and material. It's been said, "When the student is ready, the teacher appears." And the teacher, your own Inner Glutton, has been with you this whole time to lead you to health and back to your whole self.

This time is different because we're not going to treat this part of us in the same critical way. We're not going to fight her, shame her, or force her. We're going to love her.

The shaming behavior pattern must end for true health to emerge. Rather than the constant inner brutality, partner with your Inner Glutton to understand what she's trying to tell you.

> There's no condemnation in Christ Jesus, but there's been plenty of condemnation within our own self.

All this to say, she has been your companion for many reasons. When she acts out, it's not because she wants to sabotage you, but it's because she's trying to help, to offer love by stuffing you with food. And like that ugly birthday gift, you're thinking, *Thanks, but no really, you shouldn't have.*

Might I ask, how is your relationship with you? How do you treat yourself when you feel you've sabotaged your efforts? Do you offer compassion to yourself? Do you treat yourself harshly by restricting? Do you make excuses and stay circling the mountain? Or can we mistake you for a UFC boxing champ?

Over time, as you learn how to do relationships with yourself, God, food, and people better, Inner Glutton transforms, and she heals from feeling shamed and unsafe. She no longer uses food to fill unmet needs. She's a loving partner with you on the journey to a whole, free, abundant life.

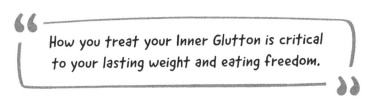

> How you treat your Inner Glutton is critical to your lasting weight and eating freedom.

And you may think you're great at relationships, but if we look closer, are you really sharing your true vulnerabilities? Or is food helping you to cope with all that mushy stuff?

As you gain greater consciousness, throughout this delightful reading experience (I hope), you'll learn patterns, behaviors, and self-talk from the Inner Glutton to prevent food fights. How you treat your Inner Glutton is critical to your lasting weight and eating freedom.

Let's learn how to love *all* of you—mistakes, love handles, warts, and all. Your Inner Glutton wants to help you learn how to love yourself. She seeks food because she's soul hungry, eating for comfort, fun, connection, and healing. She's using food to help get these needs met.

1. **Inner Glutton wants comfort.** Eating comforts. Life can be challenging, and we all need comfort. The act of eating itself with the sensations of taste, touch, sight, and smell stimulated, gives us comfort we need in life's happenstances. From the time we're babies, sucking and chewing soothes.

    Every human needs food, but when Inner Glutton is eating too much or choosing the wrong stuff, she's attempting to be comforted from a host of non-physiological needs by food. Food is and always will be a type of comfort.

And even if you don't live in the south, we know comfort foods are good for the soul but really rough on the hips. We, however, eat for comfort too frequently. And comfort isn't only at a funeral repast but in daily life. This requires intervention of the supernatural kind. How can you lean into Holy Spirit to provide comfort?

2. **Inner Glutton wants fun.** Eating is a form of fun. The average American works forty-seven hours a week according to Gallup data.[1] We wake up early to get to work and stay up late to get work done. Leisure isn't a nice-to-have part of life, it's a need. Church folk are guilty of not enough enjoyment. Some churches have so many services all throughout the week, who has time to see the world or enjoy nature?

    Fun is underrated.

    Food has been the only acceptable thing some folks have fun with. We've given up college age ideas of fun, but we still need fun. Hectic parts of life are managed better when balanced with pleasure.

    > Leisure isn't a nice-to-have part of life, it's a need.

    Enjoy family, friends, nature, and new adventures. To squeeze less pleasure out of food, we need to squeeze more pleasure out of life. The Inner Glutton is a girl (or guy) who just wants to have fun, but fun ends up in a brawl with mug shots. Her search to feel better, for stimulation, starts with a slice and quickly leads to a whole pizza.

    Sadly, she gets amnesia the next day. Is your life too much work and not enough play? Where else can you gather pleasure instead of from food? What leisure activities can you enjoy without living around food? What hobbies can you develop?

3. **Inner Glutton wants connection.** Inner Glutton perceives food as love. According to Maslow's hierarchy of needs, every human has a need for family love, relationships, and belonging. But, what if it's unsafe or difficult to connect with others?

> **We just feel safer with food than siblings, parents, spouses, or colleagues.**

What if she feels lonely and has no one to talk to? Eating may be more reliable than people. We need others to listen and understand us. We just feel safer with food than siblings, parents, spouses, or colleagues. We try to love ourselves—only eating love is short lived because it's followed quickly by guilt. Guilt is an alarm that says the love we're trying to offer isn't real love at all.

Inner Glutton wants your love, your friendship. But you've been so frustrated with her activities you may not realize how much you condemn, judge, hurt, or criticize her. You hold a part of yourself in contempt.

Our constant attack toward unfavorable food behaviors causes more unfavorable food behaviors. It sparks a rebellion from your

> **Give yourself the gift of being your own good friend.**

Inner Glutton because you're not listening. Give yourself the gift of being your own good friend. Be kind, loving, encouraging, and forgive yourself, especially when you fail. How can you be a better friend to you? What real friendships can you develop?

4. **Your Inner Glutton wants your healing.** We eat and distract ourselves from the emotions we need to feel and identity we need to heal. Every time Inner Glutton acts up, there's a chance to learn who you are and what's eating you.

   Your Inner Glutton has insight to help you to grow beyond any part of your identity that's confused, broken, hurt, or damaged from an upbringing where you were not emotionally heard, validated, approved, encouraged, or honored for the unique, fearfully and wonderfully made, marvelous soul that God made you to be (Psalm 139:14).

A shame based identity is a false identity because it lives in lies about who you are. Your real self is hidden and wants to come out of hiding. Your Inner Glutton can help you discover your truth by bringing out your identity into a restored, whole, authentic you. Your authentic you doesn't have this struggle or excess soul, body, or spiritual weight.

Let's work with our Inner Glutton to see beyond the tactics into our true heart to heal every empty place we try to fill. When Inner Glutton emerges, seek healing and ask yourself, "Am I being the real me?" or "What's on my heart?"

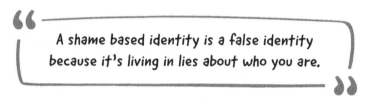

> A shame based identity is a false identity because it's living in lies about who you are.

We'll discuss Diet Nut in subsequent chapters. For now, can you see how much your Inner Glutton wants to help you gain comfort, fun, connection, and healing?

The Unmet Needs of Inner Glutton

Unmet needs drive our sabotaging behaviors. Essentially, unmet needs trigger Inner Glutton. At the core of our destructive behavior is an unmet need we're trying to fill. But the hole in our soul cannot be filled with the wrong filler. It's like filling a car up with water in the tank. It won't move right, and no amount you pour into the tank will make it go.

An unmet need must be acknowledged or met. A need is not, and probably won't ever be, a bag of M&M's®. This may satisfy an addicted, physiological need for sugar, chocolate, or fat but not a sincere heart need.

Common scenarios that trigger Inner Glutton:

- Your spouse yells at you when you need to feel heard. Inner Glutton is there for you with gummy bears.
- Your boss cuts you off in a work meeting when you need validation. Inner Glutton soothes your upset with ice cream.
- Your money isn't covering bills when you need financial security. Inner Glutton provides chocolate to cope with the stress of lack of resources.

In these examples, a need had to be acknowledged. When Inner Glutton is on the verge of sabotage, ask yourself, "What do I need?" Then, acknowledge that. Simply say, "I need connection." Give this need to the Holy Spirit, and He will comfort you and provide ideas to get that need met, such as "Call Cindy" or "Pray." This process is almost so simple it's silly. But it works.

All your need *needs* is to be acknowledged. If not, your heart's cry is stuffed down with chips and guac. As you learn, observe, and seek what's underneath your Inner Glutton's episodes, you'll get to know yourself and your needs.

> A need is not, and probably won't ever be, a bag of M&M's.

What Do You Need?

The Inner Glutton struggles to get needs met in a healthy way because she learned early in life that she wasn't worthy of getting her needs met. When we learn this through subtle and overt rejection from caregivers, we stop relying on other people to meet our needs.

To meet our needs, Inner Glutton resorts to what she knows best: eating too much, choosing the wrong stuff, not choosing the right stuff, and neglecting herself.

> We've become dependent on food as an extension of our false identity, centered around shaming and guilting ourselves.

Only it doesn't satisfy.

We've become dependent on food as an extension of our false identity, centered around shaming and guilting ourselves.

We have dependency needs that we've felt too ashamed or undeserving to have met. Peek at the dependency needs below and ponder how your unmet needs have triggered you to overeat.

Self-Value	Stimulation	Socially Healthy Primary Caretakers	Structure	Security	Stroking
• You feel you matter • You're taken seriously • Sense of being for oneself • Sense of self • Being different	• Pleasure/pain • Fun • Excitement • Challenge • Play	• Mirroring/echoing • Affirmation of feelings, needs, time, and drives • Interpersonal bridge • Identification • Need to nurture • Significant relationship	• Direction • Modeling • Boundaries • Predictability • Having limits set	• Medical care • Enough food • Protection • Clothing • Shelter	• Attention • Being recognized • Being held and touched • Encouragement • Praise • Warmth

Figure 14.2 Basic Dependency Needs in Adult Life [Adopted from *Healing the Shame that Binds You* by John Bradshaw] [2]

In addition to dependency needs, consider Maslow's Hierarchy of Needs. Abraham Maslow originally created the Hierarchy of Needs Theory in 1943. He classified human needs into three areas: physiological needs (body), psychological needs (soul), and self-actualization (spirit).

If the physiological needs—food, shelter, and water—aren't met, it may be difficult to aspire to the higher oriented spirituality of self-actualization (God given potential) or transcendence (helping others get free).[3]

Which of your needs do you have difficulty getting met? Place those needs before God in prayer as we continue to gain more understanding about them.

Figure 14.3 Maslow's Hierarchy of Needs[4]

The Observation Assignment

The most important action you can do right now is become conscious to your Inner Glutton's unmet needs and triggers. Observe your Inner Glutton. Note your observations. Track his episodes. Like a detective, look for clues on your unmet needs—the when, why, what, and how he is eating.

The art of observation is first becoming conscious to the part of you that sabotages. Observation leads to exploration. Exploration leads to understanding. Understanding leads to new strategies. Through observation, we can learn to mitigate causes and their effects.

Be sure to log your observations over the next several weeks so that you'll be more alert to your Inner Glutton and Diet Nut's cycles of destruction.

As a lifelong practice:

- Observe how you respond to your eating mistakes. Pay attention to how you speak to yourself. Are you loving or critical? Kind or mean?

- Observe events, feelings, and situations that led to eating mistakes. Watch what triggers an overeating episode. Notice Diet Nut's reactions when your Inner Glutton has acted out.

- Observe your food patterns in greater detail. What foods spark obsessive eating, down moods, food cravings, or feeling ashamed of your body?

You'll get aha! moments as you observe and log your findings about your Inner Glutton. As you learn over time, he'll heal.

Like Sam realized, "My Inner Glutton was really active on Friday night after work. For as long as I can remember, I tend to overeat on Friday nights. Hmm, maybe my Inner Glutton's exhausted from the week. It seems I need fun and connection to balance out work, but I find food instead. I can plan something to look forward to on Friday nights."

Or Yasmeen recognized, "My Inner Glutton is very active after conversations with my uncle. What is it about our conversation topics that makes me eat after our calls? He always talks negatively about my mother, and I want to say something, but [aha! moment] I'm eating what I want to say!"

"I can journal out what I want to say, and the next time I speak with him, I'll be honest." Yasmeen tried this and she noticed she didn't eat so much after their calls. It was difficult to be honest, but her observation helped her gather insight and correct a piece of the weight and eating puzzle.

As you become more conscious, your whole self partners with your Inner Glutton and Diet Nut. Observation is the main daily task because we're in the process of becoming more aware to who and what we're hiding under our false sense of identity. As we move along, we'll continue to build on this foundation. Because, there's an entrenched fear to overcome to heal your Inner Glutton.

The fear of the Whole Self.

REFLECT & SHARE

1. Have you felt shame around your needs?

_____

_____

_____

2. What need did your Inner Glutton want acknowledged last time he/she acted up?

_____

_____

_____

3. How can you offer more love and support to yourself when you mess up?

_____

_____

_____

CHAPTER 15

THE FEAR OF THE WHOLE SELF

There's a certain truth why we call love handles, love handles.

Inner Glutton and Diet Nut are a part of the bound self, the part of you bound in fear. As a foundation to lasting freedom, the spirit of fear is the root of the saga of weight and eating troubles. To heal the drama within we increase in love as we decrease in fear.

How we use food is like a measuring stick to how much we stand in love. When we use food in a way that reveals the body, more love is at work. When we use food in a way that hides the body, more fear is at work.

Some of us may not hide in weight but in berating thoughts about our body image, or never feeling skinny or muscular enough. This too is fear in operation.

Our gluttony, our obsession, is a fear of not having enough food, love, or comfort. The body of your dreams is waiting to be revealed. It's already there. You're in that handsome body now. Excess weight hides our most attractive body, which means it also hides our most vibrant, fearless self.

Surprisingly, the battle isn't with bread, it's between love and fear. The whole self and the bound self. Truth and lies.

The heart of weight and eating psychology is our transition from fear to love, from self-harm to a self-love lifestyle, from carnal to spiritual, and from staunch legalism evidenced by calorie counting or strict diets to balanced grace. We're in a transformation process, and God is using your food and weight struggles to do it.

> **The battle isn't with bread, it's between love and fear.**

The Root of Weight & Eating Bondage

In all bondage is torment and fear. There's one dominant fear we all deal with in our transformation process: the fear of the whole self. Our whole self adopts the fullness of our identity.

> **We're in a transformation process, and God is using your food and weight struggles to do it.**

Fear involves torment. "There is no fear in love; but perfect love casts out fear, because fear involves torment. But he who fears has not been made perfect in love" (1 John 4:18). We all know weight and eating bondage is torment—from obsessing about food to shaming our bodies. When there's torment, we know fear took up residence.

But fear of what?

Fear of our whole self. We not only deny godly power, but we deny our own power of God in us as well. We deny our own godliness, the healthy part of us, operating in the power of the Spirit.

Our healthiest self is a part of that light and love. In health, we're shiny, vibrant, and bright. We have energy, overflow in joy, and abound in love. We're a magnet for attracting people. We feel our best because in health we are our best. We're scared of this. We know: "For God has not given us a spirit of fear, but of power, love and a sound mind" (2 Timothy 1:7).

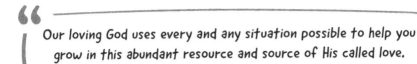

> Our loving God uses every and any situation possible to help you grow in this abundant resource and source of His called love.

God is love (1 John 4:8). The fruit of the spirit is love (Galatians 5:22). We want to better embody the spirit of God. We want Him to flow through us. This requires a version of you that you've been previously afraid to receive. Our loving God uses every and any situation possible to help you grow in this abundant resource and source of His called love.

Love is the prescription for fear, shame, and guilt. Love is the currency of the kingdom of God. And love matters more than anything else. As Paul put it, we can do many things, but if love isn't at the root and the source, then it's in vain because it lacks the agape, unconditional, abundant source that is God, Who is love (1 Corinthians 13:1–13; John 4:8).

The Purpose of Torment

On the other hand, "torment is a source of vexation, infliction of torture, extreme pain or anguish of body and/or mind."[1] Yet, we know God is not in torment but that "all things work together for good to those who love God and are called according to *His* purpose" (Romans 8:28).

The goal of torment is to distract us from God given purpose, relationship with Him, other people, and momentum. It's to delay your mission. To block you from finding your mission. It's to prevent you from the joy of your current sphere of influence.

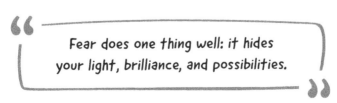

> Fear does one thing well: it hides your light, brilliance, and possibilities.

Weight and eating torment is the smokescreen over our true greatness and power in the Holy Spirit. We glorify God when we choose to walk whole, healed, and delivered, not in our comforts of walking broken, hurt, and bound.

Fear does one thing well: it hides your light, brilliance, and possibilities. To expose ourselves in the form of reduced fat exteriors isn't safe. We're scared of who we are on the other side. In fear is every negative emotion. Shame, hate, guilt, and jealousy are all roommates in the mansion of fear.

Fear of the Whole Self

Fear of the whole self was identified by spirituality teacher Miriam Williamson in her book *A Return to Love*. She said in beautiful prose, "Our greatest fear is not that we are inadequate, but that we are powerful beyond measure. It is our light, not our darkness, that frightens us." [2]

Author and Pastor Chad Dedmon illustrated this point well. One night, while dreaming, he saw himself looking in the mirror. He looked but his reflection back was distorted, and the mirrors looked like that of a haunted house. His skin was drooped, eyes mismatched, clothes disheveled, and hands mangled. He realized this gross image in the mirror was the image of how he saw himself.

Then a light pierced the room, and the mirrors changed.

Light gathered the mirrors to show the truth to Pastor Chad of how Jesus saw him. He sensed the light was Jesus, and Pastor Chad couldn't look. The image of how God saw him was too beautiful to look at fully.

Instead he raised his forearm above his elbow, staring away one second and curious the next. He was fearful of his own beauty, awe, and wonder of his God created, whole, beautiful self.

He'd rather go back to the horrifying image as that distorted image felt comfortable. But, because Light pierced through the old man and penetrated love deep into the soul of his son, Pastor Chad was able to withstand his godliness.

When he awoke, he cried, realizing he encountered God's love. And it would be God's love that would heal his identity.[3]

We fear our whole, vibrant, beautiful, good self, and hide under weight and poor habits to somehow reduce the greatness of the fact that we're children of God and a glowing expression of Him.

We've been confused about our identities as children of God. Instead of shining our lights fully, free of weight and eating turmoil, we stay stuck in failure with our attention on this one area of our lives that we can't seem to grasp, whereas many other strengths go uncelebrated. We are more than our weight problems.

These antics of trying to lose weight then sabotage with food reflects the lack of love we have within. We fear we can't get or sustain healthier bodies. We couldn't handle the success, attention, adoration, expectations, and responsibilities of being free.

We don't want to be seen. To shine is to risk failure or rejection. But it's our light God calls us to shine.

> To shine is to risk failure or rejection.

From Bound to Free

Healing the Shame that Binds You is a celebrated book on the topic of shame by psychology leader John Bradshaw. He said, "A sense of identity forms the foundation for a healthy adult love relationship." A healthy sense of identity is also the foundation for a healthy relationship with food and your body. He goes on to say, "A toxically shamed person is divided within himself and must create a false-self cover to hide (and validate) his sense of being flawed and defective."[4]

In other words, because the bound self believes, "I'm defective, broken, worthless, wrong, and inadequate," it operates accordingly and is bound in the lie of believing these things, thinking it's who she is.

The bound self keeps us stuck in the shame and guilt cycle as well as the behavioral patterns that validates feeling unworthy and guilty. The bound self rejects receiving the Father's unconditional love. Because shame says, *Who am I to be loved by a deeply loving God? Who am I to be in His presence? Who am I to be set free?*

This shame based identity crisis happens when we don't know who we are. Because of not knowing who we are, we settle for what is or has been instead of reaching for new ways to evolve and redefine ourselves in alignment with truth. Because of not knowing who we are, we don't believe God can or will help us. We're stuck in unbelief.

The whole self is a healed, firm, redefined identity. It's a belief about you that aligns with God's truth about you. You're free to be joyful, happy, sincere, accepting, beautiful, and strong. The whole self is the development of the fruit of the Spirit in your life and soul. It's your spiritual you.

> "The bound self rejects receiving the Father's unconditional love.

The key here is we're both bound and whole at the same time. And as we decrease in fear, we increase in love. The less Inner Glutton acts up, the more whole self grows.

Healing the Bound Self

Cynthia came into my therapy office frustrated about her weight.

"Jendayi, I just don't understand why I can't make progress. It's so frustrating!" Her shoulders slouched on the red fabric sofa.

"Cynthia, let's take a look at what's going on inside. How would you describe the relationship between the part of you that wants to be healthier and the part of you that doesn't?" I gently inquired, leaning in.

"One part of me keeps sabotaging myself. I hear myself saying you'll always be sick and tired, and you'll always be on medications so why bother? Just eat whatever you want!" Tears swelled in her eyes as this lie came to light.

I gave her a soft pillow to hold onto as I instructed her to close her eyes and get comfortable.

"Cynthia, ask that part of you that feels harsh, why it's there?"

A deep sob emerged, her mascara running down her cheeks.

"I don't believe in myself. I don't believe I can do it. I can't do anything right is what my mom always told me." She took the next few minutes to process, sobbing quietly. I asked her, "Will you ask this part of you to work with you going forward?

"Will you work with me and believe in me?" She inquired and then responded after she sensed her inner wisdom, "Yes!"

I asked, "How can she help you instead of criticizing?"

She asked, "Will you help me instead by encouraging me and letting me know I can do things right? Will you help me by saying you can do it Cynthia, or Cynthia, you're good enough?" As she made the request to her Inner Glutton, she unified this division of herself. Her face brightened, and a crooked smile emerged from her pink lips.

This was the start for Cynthia to create peace between her bound self that was sabotaging her and her whole self.

Let me summarize in daily life terms. You buy a boatload of vegetables with the intention of eating all the nutrients your body could ingest. Instead, you go the easy route throughout the week. You order from your favorite Chinese place, go out to dinner with friends, get pizza for the kids, and before you know it, those vegetables in the fridge are moldy with a stench. Why is it you intend to do such good but end up wasting pricey produce?

The crux of every human being: we have a carnal nature, that is a self-harming nature, and it lives in us by the very law of being human.

Love is the answer to the inner turmoil. When we're in wholeness, we operate from our whole self. We act out of unconditional love, acceptance, happiness, peace, contentment, kindness, appreciation, gratitude, and security.

The whole self believes it's worthy, capable, perfectly imperfect, and good enough. This relationship we have with self must find a place of unity, partnership, and support. In other words, the love is the healing balm to your fear.

> " When we're in wholeness, we operate from our whole self. "

Sin Is Not a Four-Letter Word

Oftentimes people shiver at the word sin, as if they've got the cooties or just heard a pastor utter a four-letter word from the pulpit. The word sin has been used like a hammer, beating nonbelievers into hell and damnation. It causes some ministry leaders of today to neglect being upfront about sin altogether, leaving congregants struggling and unrepentant.

But, what if the word sin wasn't so emotionally charged with visions of lakes of fire and brimstone? What if sin indicated our fear of the whole self?

Sin is perceived by our Father in Heaven in the same way a parent is grieved when they see their child using street drugs or hanging out with the wrong crowd.

Jesus advocated, "Repent, [turn away from self-harm], for the kingdom of heaven is at hand" (Matthew 4:17). Jesus came to free us of the law of sin and death by His salvation and our willing obedience toward His ways over our own. It is by grace through faith alone that we are saved (Ephesians 2:8).

Sin is self-harm. As James says, "Therefore, to him who knows to do good and does not do *it*, to him it is sin" (James 4:17). And Proverbs 8:36a says, "He who sins against me (wisdom/Lord) wrongs His own soul." To damage the body is sin. Sin is failure or missing the mark. The mark is the Word of God or God's teaching and instruction. Living in God's love and light, we don't intentionally sin.

Sin is an indicator of fear. Sin is bound by shame, doubt, and unbelief. Many self-help books are truly sin-help books. We struggle, and we need God's help with our sin to heal the fear and shame causing it.

> **Sin is perceived by our Father in Heaven in the same way a parent is grieved when they see their child using street drugs or hanging out with the wrong crowd.**

When we self-harm, like a rebellious child, we harm God. And we harm others who witness our pain because we as a human species are interconnected and impact one another.

A dear colleague was morbidly obese. To the point I wondered if she got up to go to the bathroom or if she dressed herself. She had whole cakes in her office and ate them all too. She sat behind her desk and ate all day, making strange frog like sounds from her throat randomly. As a supervising counselor she oversaw counseling students. Her death affected her family, her students, her colleagues, and others—just as it had hurt everyone around her to see her destroy herself.

The autopsy report said the cause of death was cancer, but cancer has evidence that it's a result of eating processed foods and toxic ingredients. Researchers put it this way, "Worldwide, we estimate that 481,000 or 3.6 percent of all new cancer cases in adults in 2012 were attributable to high BMI."[5]

Obesity isn't the cause of any death on autopsy reports. Other diseases related to obesity are such as heart disease or diabetes. We instinctively know that sin, over time, when it's full grown, gives birth to death (James 1:15).

Sin is self-induced negligence causing grief, injury, and death to the spirit, soul, and body. The word sin gets a bad rap. But it's followed by one of the most beautiful words, repentance.

To repent is to say, "God, I've mismanaged myself. I've agreed with death. I've agreed with darkness. I want to agree with you. I want to agree with life. I want to be worthy of life. I choose life."

To repent is to turn from death to life. To repent is to take a spiritual shower. Ultimately, to repent is to say no to an identity rooted in self-harm to one rooted in love—deep love for the Father and yourself as His creation. When we truly turn away, because we've realized our self-harm, we shift our old man from that which agreed with death to our new man which agrees with life, body, soul, spirit care, and love.

To repent is to take a spiritual shower.

To love anyone, including ourselves, requires loving God. When we open up to greater love, we can receive the grace and healing power needed to love ourselves.

Bottom line: you must learn to love yourself.

A measurement of growth for this is the SEAS self-esteem inventory. See Non-Edible Goodies. Get a score for your level of self-esteem so you can witness how much you'll grow over time into someone who really loves who God made you.

Break Down Fear Walls

We'll need to break down fear walls to increase in love. Fear walls are constructs that create a barrier both to and from our naked soul. They're built by beliefs and interpretations from life's traumas and experiences. Fear walls are built when we've felt unsafe, unprotected, or undervalued for we were. And instead our value was placed in what we've looked like, what we've had, or what we could do.

Fear walls cause us to hide our real self. We can hide anywhere. In our bodies, work, minds, addictions, schedules, emotions, in people, appearances, education, money, and more. Walls create an unconscious push away effect, pushing away the threat of pain and the ability to receive love at the same time.

Fear of the whole self is exposed as we evaluate a few areas. Every time we go for a change, our subconscious evaluates the reflection questions coming up. When these questions don't check out to be safe, we won't be able to sustain the change for long. The fear of the whole self needs some time to allow you and your body to come out of hiding.

And if you're a normal weight but feel bound in your negative thoughts about your body or still binge with food, consider what's on the other side of letting this sabotaging mental behavior go. And step into a greater you with acceptance of your body, ambition, power, attractiveness, or all of the above.

This journey to your whole self is a work in progress.

But this time is different. This time you're facing you, not just your thighs, but all of you. Thank God for the struggle! Thank God for the extra poundage! Thank God for the many attempts to heal this issue. Thank God for revealing it all.

Because of it, you are being made more perfect in love.

> **You are being made more perfect in love.**

REFLECT & SHARE

1. What does it mean for you to step into your whole self?

2. What criticisms do you fear receiving as you step into your whole self?

3. What losses could you experience when you step into your whole self?

4. What insecurities would be difficult to cope with when you step into your whole self?

5. How does it feel to rejoice for your weight and eating struggles?

CHAPTER 16

CHUBBOLOGY
WHY WE SELF-PROTECT WITH WEIGHT

Losing weight is easy; it's allowing it to go for good that's hard.

As you step into your whole self, you'll see fitting your soul is more important than those skinny jeans. Who knew? We're going to explore threats to our weight release in what I call Chubbology.

Chubbology
(noun) Chubb-ba-lo-gy
the made up psychological study of why we use weight for self-protection

Like our Inner Glutton's there to help us in strange ways, same is true about our weight. Our *chubby suit* is here for the greater good, but we hate wearing it. We may not *want* the weight or the struggle, but we *need* the weight and the struggle to protect our soul for good reasons.

The depth of intelligence in our psyche ensures that if we didn't have a reason to use weight to self-protect, we wouldn't. This gives us hope for weight release when these reasons resolve in our soul.

Losing weight is easy; it's allowing it to go for good that's hard. Excess body weight serves as a form of self-protection. It's nature's natural handgun, armed and ready against any perceived threats to our soul's safety.

We can wear a chubby suit to look less attractive to repel the opposite sex because we feel threatened by our sexuality. We can wear our chubby suit as a barrier from being too close to someone because we don't want to risk our hearts getting hurt again. We can wear it to stay stuck so the real us won't risk failure. We can wear a chubby suit to feel the physical affection missing in our life.

Ever get duped by a prank-can that you open? Our weight release is like a prank-can with a jelly bean exterior. It looks good on the outside. Then suddenly, out jumps a paper snake. We gasp and want to put the lid back on. The snake is the threat triggering fear we didn't know was there or we weren't prepared to handle.

The lid is the weight we've released. And just like that prank-can full of surprise, but packed in a jelly bean exterior, we're frightened. In our chub rationale, we keep our excess weight to protect our vulnerable, unsafe soul.

Try to recall how many times you've both gained and lost more than twenty pounds in your life? Chances are you were confronted with a threat that your soul wasn't ready to handle.

The 7 Threats of Why We Self-Protect with Weight

We can diet all we want, but in the end, if we don't deal with threats to releasing weight, all that's lost will be found again. On the flipside, we can become more accepting of our weight because of the purpose it serves.

A trigger is what sparks a series of actions or self-sabotaging behaviors.

This chapter is focused on *chubbological triggers*, of which the soul experiences a perceived threat to its safety, causing weight to ricochet. Let's look at the seven threats and corresponding fears that make us use weight as a protective barrier. We'll face specific fears we've been hiding in.

I'll warn you, this chapter can stir up tough emotions. Notice your emotional body's responses as you read. If you start thinking about your favorite binge foods, take a deep breath and lean into the Holy Spirit for comfort. If that doesn't work, skip to the next chapter until you're ready. Or go to Chapter 18 to practice an Emotional Fitness Workout™. Each threat may not resonate but rank the ones that do in order of resonance.

CHUBBOLOGICAL TRIGGERS	THREATS
Unwanted Attention	#1 Attractiveness
Unbridled Sexual Lust	#2 Sexual Lust
Vulnerability	#3 Emotional Intimacy
Rejection	#4 Criticism
Loss of Self-Concept	#5 Self-Concept
Loss or Abandonment	#6 Other People's Insecurity
Dealing with Emotional Pain	#7 Deep Life Disappointments

Threat #1 – Attractiveness
Chubbological Trigger – Unwanted Attention

Nancy just finished a successful six weeks at Weight Watchers. Proud of her efforts to drop fifteen pounds, she decided to go out and celebrate with a girlfriend. They went to the local dance school's ballroon party night.

Nancy attracted a creepy guy who insisted she dance with him.

"Hey beautiful, do you salsa?" he asked, as he placed his hand on her lower back.

"Yes, but …," her words too shy to permeate the loud music.

"It's my lucky day," he said close to her ear. Latin drums blasted the speakers as he swiftly moved into salsa dancing with Nancy.

After a couple songs she mustered the courage to tell him she had to go to the ladies' room. She and her girlfriend grabbed their purses and snuck out the back door.

The next day, Nancy felt funny, but she couldn't put her finger on why. But she did manage to put her fingers all over chocolate bars, and she ate a few daily. Over the next few weeks, Nancy regained all the weight she lost and then some.

Nancy thought she wanted to lose weight, but in losing weight she gained male attention. Digging deeper, she had past sexual trauma. Because of this trauma, she had a tendency to enter into abusive relationships. Her soul wasn't ready to release the weight because releasing the weight gained her attention from men she wasn't equipped to handle.

Intimidated by aggressive men, she didn't have the confidence yet to state her boundaries or preferences. Once Nancy's attractiveness was tested, her army of fat stampeded right back to defend her.

Nancy's scared of unwanted attention. Nancy pondered, *Will he force me to do something I don't want to do? Will he hurt me?*

Probable Causes of the Fear of Unwanted Attention

- We've been sexually abused, molested, or assaulted in some way.
- We've been in physically abusive relationships.
- We feel nervous or intimidated by the opposite sex.
- We've been ashamed of secret, same-sex sexual abuse.
- We don't have established boundaries with the opposite sex.

Reflection Question: Have you fully resolved your past sexual abuse?

With some of these probable causes, it only makes sense to hide in your chubby suit to avoid attention that you're not ready for. We use weight to protect ourselves from the unwanted attention our attractiveness can bring.

Unwanted attention is the kind you don't know how to handle. When our beauty or handsomeness has harmed us, we can hide in a chubby suit because we don't know how to deal with attention from the opposite sex.

We can use our bigness to feel more powerful against threats to our physical safety when we've had negative sexual attention in the past such as molestation, rape, assault, or incest. Studies show twenty percent of females and five to ten percent of males recall sexual abuse from childhood.[1] An analysis of 57,000 females reported twice as much food addiction with a history of childhood sexual abuse than those with no history.[2]

To resolve sexual abuse requires regular professional therapeutic care. In a therapeutic relationship, you're empowered to create boundaries, use your voice without being intimidated by others, and heal deep grief. You're not alone. Past abuse is the biggest threat in the weight and eating equation.

> **We can hide in a chubby suit because we don't know how to deal with attention from the opposite sex.**

A weight loss doctor, Dr. Wendy Scinta, in Manlius, New York, says she now includes questions about abuse when clients utilize her services, and she started a group therapy session because the majority, especially of those with 100 or more pounds to lose, have tragic abuse stories in their past.[3] This doctor understands the chubbological threat, and she knew clients had to deal with their past trauma before they could see lasting results.[4] Research shows that post-traumatic stress, like sexual abuse, leads to obesity.[5]

Take a deep breath. I've had my share of sexual abuse, too. I can empathize. You'll know when an issue is fully resolved because there's no anger, tears, or emotional charge around it. You can talk about it freely, and it becomes a testimony to share with others in your life.

You'll know it's resolved when you've forgiven all involved parties, including yourself. When resolved, you've also overcome toxic beliefs, such as unworthiness, self-hatred, toxic shame or guilt, and any gender related bitterness that took hold during sexual abuse like man or woman hating.

The extraordinary, Joyce Meyer is an exemplary example of healing and wholeness from traumatic sexual abuse all throughout her childhood. I love hearing her stories of restoration. Consider her books as well as the *Victim to Victory* manual for healing sexual abuse by Brenda Clark-Dandridge.

You are clean. You are safe. And you have new discernment you didn't have when you were abused. You have new tools, skills, friends, and community. And if you don't, you can create a life to feel safe and protected.

Threat #2 – Sexual Lust
Chubbological Trigger – Unbridled Sexual Lust

Jim was a lady's man in his earlier days when he played football for his high school team. Years later, he struggled with seventy extra pounds. He pushed memories away of being too sexual with girls and cheating on his girlfriends with football fans. In marriage, his wife was unhappy with his weight. He lost and gained weight several times in their twenty years of marriage.

Jim feared his own sexual lust would be set loose and he'd risk losing his family. Each time he lost weight, he'd get flirtatious attention from women.

He thought, *What if I look like I did back then? Would I act the same? I could make the horrible mistake of cheating on my wife and lose my family. Oh God, would I be a heathen again?*

Judy loved God with all of her heart. She, like many God seekers, attended programs to learn about God and understand who she was in Christ. Over time, her spiritual transformation and learning allowed her to release forty pounds.

Then Reggie came along.

Smitten by his charm and dark features, she struggled with her desire for him and her desire to keep her sexual purity. After a while of entertaining her on-again, off-again relationship with Reggie, her sexual lust overtook her, followed by his complete rejection.

Her mistake caused her to regain the forty pounds and then some.

Her life regained traction, but it was difficult to cope with her own sexual lust.

In her past, she struggled with promiscuity and never learned how to relate to men in a non-sexual way. Reggie was her first relationship she had in many years, and it proved her chubbology right.

She pondered, *I can't handle the opposite sex. How do I interact in a plutonic way with men instead of being so physical?* And deeper, *what else can I give if I gave myself fully and was still rejected?*

Cecille flirted with an ex on social media. One thing led to another, and she and her ex met up one night at the bar. After several drinks, her inhibitions left, and lust aggressively took over. Ashamed the next day, she confessed to her husband what she'd done. Shame filled her. And weight followed. After two years of marital counseling since the affair, Cecille struggled to let the fifty pounds she gained, go.

"I don't trust myself," Cecille confessed in my office. "What if I cheat again?"

"Ask the weight why it's there," I said.

"I think my weight protects me from myself. I guess at fifty pounds heavier I can't get into too much trouble," she laughed.

Cecille knew at some level her weight repelled sexual advances, as her physical body, needed self-protection from the threat of her sexual lust and the depth of pain the sexual tension had caused in her marriage.

She loved her husband and didn't want to commit another act of adultery. However, her beauty, her physical body, felt safe in her chubby suit because it suppressed the sexual part of herself.

Her internal sense of self didn't trust her own ability to stay adultery free. She wondered, *Could I control myself if I lost weight? What if a man I'm attracted to likes me back? What would I do?*

Probable Causes of the Fear of Unbridled Sexual Lust

- We've harmed another with adultery or cheating in the past.
- We've suppressed our own sexuality.

- We are challenged to trust our own sexual self-control because of previous mistakes.
- We have unresolved sexual self-abuse like chronic masturbation or promiscuity.
- We've been too physical too soon in past relationships.

Reflection Question: Have you reconciled your unbridled sexual lust and the damages your lust has caused?

Watch for my upcoming book, *Stupid Sex!* I'll provide more practical advice to work through sexual history and its impact on relationships. A trusted counselor can work with you to talk through any part of your soul bound in shame about your sexual past.

Over time, you learn how to trust your sexual self-control as your whole self becomes firm.

I strongly believe lust is lust. If sexual lust is unresolved, the spirit of lust will transfer to another area like decadent food.

Be bold. Heal your sexual history.

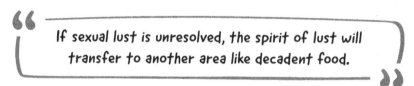

> If sexual lust is unresolved, the spirit of lust will transfer to another area like decadent food.

Threat #3 – Emotional Intimacy [Romantic Love]
Chubbological Trigger – Vulnerability

Bob loved to cook. And it was something he longed to share with his wife. He'd lost weight to find Renee, but as soon as he married Renee, he was cooking alright. Within months of the marriage, they were both buying two sizes larger of clothing.

"You've got to stop cooking so many delicious foods. I'm getting fat," Renee said. "I want to be able to fit in my clothes, and it's the second time I'm buying a larger size since I met you!"

"You look great to me, honey," Bob said, mixing the dough for an apple pie as he winked in her direction.

"I don't feel great to me. And you've gained weight, too. I really don't want to be the chubby couple," she laughed, amidst her seriousness. "Babe, I just don't want to set this kind of stage for our children."

Bob felt the same way. But he cooked with her because it was easier to sit and eat than it was for him to sit and talk. He too felt plagued with frustration about his own weight and eating struggles. But marriage was both exciting and uncomfortable. It brought out insecurities of being abandoned.

He wondered, *What if she leaves me? What if she cheats on me? What if she uses my shortcomings as ammunition?*

Katie went through a devastating divorce. Her husband left her with their four children for her to raise on her own. And he went to live in another state with another woman. Food was her comfort from an early age but amplified after abandonment. She decided to get gastric bypass surgery after her youngest went to college.

She quickly slimmed down from a size 25 to 14. Elated, she thought she'd online date to find love again. After her first dinner date with a guy she liked, she came home and chowed down on the doggie bag something fierce.

Liking someone was a threat to Katie. Her mind wrestled with, *What if he only likes me because I'm slim? What if he pretends to love me like my ex did before he left us? Will he call when he says he will? Will he leave me when he gets to know me?*

Probable Causes of the Fear of Vulnerability

- We were emotionally and or physically neglected or abandoned as a child.
- We carry deep shame about who we are or where we come from.
- We believe a lie that we can't be loved for who we are.
- We've experienced a hard loss of love in the past and resist opening our hearts again.

- We fear getting close to others in relationship because they could use our weaknesses as ammunition to hurt us.
- We're not ready to attract a romantic relationship.

Reflection Question: Have you resolved your ability to handle emotional intimacy?

Intimacy, or in-to-me-see, is a sense of closeness when we feel safe enough to be emotionally vulnerable, seen, heard, and known, especially with someone we are attracted to or in a close relationship with.

Much like my increase in cookie consumption when I fell in love with my (now ex) husband, vulnerability caused me to use cookies to help me cope with the threat of heartbreak. I had no exposure to healthy relationship examples, only divorces. Naturally, I didn't feel safe to be vulnerable because it wasn't modeled.

Our chubby suit protects us from the threat of romantic love and intimacy because we use it to reduce our internal sense of attractiveness. Hiding inside of our chubby suit protects us from love getting in and breaking our heart.

The downside is being fearful of love also prevents our love from escaping out and creating the life we've always wanted. When we've not had an upbringing where we were safe to be emotionally vulnerable, we wonder if someone could love us how we are.

We can reduce weight to snag a spouse, but the weight is regained because we haven't learned the skills needed to have an emotionally safe relationship. A relationship that allows you and your partner to be himself or herself is ideal. Together you can heal and grow whole as individuals and as a couple. A lack of emotional safety and vulnerability stems from emotional abuse in the past.

> Hiding inside of our chubby suit protects us from love getting in and breaking our heart.

Emotional abuse has a high correlation with obesity and using food. In our first Whole & Free Health course, 84 percent suffered from past emotional and verbal abuse as opposed to 50 percent who suffered with physical abuse.[6]

Emotional abuse is any prolonged time you've felt mistrusted, wrongly accused, ignored, manipulated to feel guilty, or provoked to anger intentionally by someone you should've been able to trust.

We don't feel safe to share in abusive environments. In your own world, you don't have to worry about your heart being exposed or harmed, nor about your dysfunctions harming anyone else. However, within intimate relationships, our insecure secrets are on display, causing a fear of vulnerability.

To be vulnerable is to be in a place open to possible attack, scorn, or ridicule.[7] To be emotionally vulnerable is to open our hearts, hand it to someone else for good keeping, and risk them throwing it in the street only for it to get run over by the 6 o'clock city bus. But be encouraged, our God is the Healer of the broken hearted.

We're to learn from our broken hearts. We learn to open our heart to a wider space of love to handle vulnerability. We're to know we're safe to keep our hearts open 24:7, like a 7-Eleven.

Threat #4 – Criticism
Chubbological Trigger – Rejection

Tina went to her family barbeque. She felt alive, healthy, and vibrant. She glowed with excitement to show everyone her transformed size 8 body. She had lost several pounds since she last saw the crew. And she never felt or looked so good. As she approached the gathering at the local park, family members looked at her, not with excitement for her transformation, but with disgust.

"Tina, you're too skinny! Come over here and eat some of these ribs," her plump grandmother said.

"That's right, Tina, I made potato salad to go with those ribs, and you'll need two helpings looking like that," her uncle chimed in laughing.

Embarrassed by the attacks on her body, Tina soothed herself with large portions of mac and cheese. Her emotions stirred a mix of grief, anger, shame, and surprise. She began her day excited and ended it bloated with both emotions and water retention.

> "We're to know we're safe to keep our hearts open 24:7, like a 7-Eleven."

Her family criticized her health progress because it meant Tina would be different. Tina's family members are for the most part obese and plagued with health ailments. Tina's slim body didn't fit in. So, the family made it their business to help her get back up to size.

Tina felt rejected by their negative evaluations of her healthy body. She thought her hard work would win their approval, instead it earned their criticism. Her family made clear attempts to bring her back to a robust waistline so that she was one of the gang.

Tina's mind obsessed, *People don't like my new body. Will they continue to reject me if I don't eat or look like them? I can't handle all the negative comments about my choices and body!*

Probable Causes of the Fear of Rejection

- We don't understand the value of criticism and feedback.
- We make the criticism about us instead of the criticizer.
- We're addicted to people's approval.
- We have an underdeveloped sense of self.
- We've not worked through body shame.
- We've been abandoned or rejected by a parent.

Reflection Question: Have you resolved your fear of rejection?

Criticism can come from those groups we need the most support from in our journey toward a whole and free life. It's scary to consider the idea of being ostracized because of your downsize. However, a part of your freedom is the release from other people's weight issues that are projected onto you as criticism.

Criticisms aren't meant to make you feel rejected or attacked. In fact, comments around your body from someone else aren't your issue.

Comments and criticisms are more about the commentator than you. So, when they criticize what they see in you, they're judging what they can't see in their own self.

Criticisms are especially hard for those who've experienced verbal abuse. Words have the power of life and death, and if words of death were spoken over you, it's difficult to feel comfortable in your soul. Naturally so, because verbally abusive caregivers outright lied to you (your soul) about who you are with their word curses. Verbal abuse creates a heightened sensitivity to negative feedback and is a threat to your soul's sense of safety.

When our own families negatively evaluate our body or choices, we feel threatened because of our human need to belong. And family is the primary place

> "Criticisms are especially hard for those who've experienced verbal abuse."

we get this need met. We need family, and we need people to love us unconditionally. So, we unconsciously sabotage positive efforts as to not ruffle family feathers and fit in.

To belong is a major factor in weight and eating because we often feel so alone and isolated in our chubby suits. To move beyond rejection is to first know you belong.

Threat #5 – Self-Concept

Chubbological Trigger – Loss of Self-Concept

Another fear of Jim's around his football glory days was his loss of self-concept or his identity that was in his size. He was known as "Big Jim" because of his naturally large physique. Two decades later after playing football, eating became his sport.

His Big Jim mantra still played in the back of his mind and was part of how he saw himself. A bigger body helped him believe he was bigger and better. On one hand, he wanted to lose weight, yet, on the other hand, he couldn't reconcile who he would be without it.

His growing body mass, belly and all, helped him to feel bigger than he felt on the inside. He thought, *Who will I be without the weight? Aren't guys supposed to be large and in charge? My husky exterior gives me a sense of power.*

"Man, Harry, is that you?! How much did you lose? You look good, bro!" John, an old friend of Harry's college study approached Harry, who was at the local park. "Come play some hoops. We need a fit guy like you on the team."

Insistent, John swatted Harry on the arm to pull him over.

Nervously, Harry pulled away and made an excuse to leave. That's when the barbeque cravings kicked in, not just for the night but for the whole week.

When he was asked to play ball because he was so "fit" looking, he knew he would make a fool of himself on the team. He was expected to be athletic, but he wasn't. His anxiety that he couldn't be who someone else wanted him to be now that he was fitter triggered his old-time baby back rib special to pop into his mind, then mouth. Harry feared the expectations that came with his slimmer body.

Harry experienced fear of other's expectations. He thought, *Why does everyone expect me to be so good at sports now? I'm not the sports guy even though I look like one now that I've lost eighty pounds. Sports isn't me.*

Probable Causes of the Fear of Loss of Self-Concept

- We've placed part of our identity in weight.
- We associate our roles with being large.
- We're unable to reconcile our roles with our body shape and size.
- We're unsure how we'll participate in our roles at a slimmer size.

- Our sense of self-esteem or bigness as a person is built into our larger size.

- We fear we will disappoint others in our new body.

- We're not sure how to be vulnerable and let others know we can't meet their expectations.

Reflection Question: What part of your self-concept is wrapped up in your body mass?

Roy Baumeister, American psychologist says, self-concept is "the individual's belief about himself or herself, including the person's attributes and who and what the self is."[8] It's necessary to test your chubby suit to see if any part of your self-concept is reinforced in a positive way and then to unravel the self-concept with new possibilities. The transition into our whole self is about us reconciling who we are chubby versus who we'll be slim.

If our self-concept has bigness as a definer, we'll have to reconcile by testing new ideas of what slim could mean for our roles and abilities. For Corinne, she needed to test a new belief that she could be both motherly and slim. For Jim, he'd need to see he's still Big Jim without being at risk for heart disease.

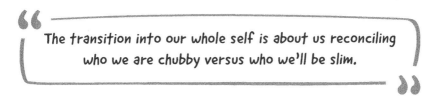

> The transition into our whole self is about us reconciling who we are chubby versus who we'll be slim.

Threat #6 – Other People's Insecurity
Chubbological Trigger – Loss or Abandonment

"Hi, honey," I said to my husband, thinking he'd think I looked awesome. I greeted him with a hug and kiss. A cold shoulder met me with a begrudged hello. Then, we argued for the next five minutes, while walking over to the event, about my skirt. My Catholic school teachers would've approved, but he did not.

"Why did you wear that? There will be a bunch of dudes there," he said.

"I thought you'd like it. I wore it to please you. And it's professional," I said, deflated.

After I spoke on health and nutrition to a group of distinguished business professionals (who unbeknownst to me were mostly men), I was met with complete silence. My husband refused to talk with me.

I was forced to mingle with my audience rather than him because he completely ignored me. *Isn't that what he didn't want?* His insecurity and fear of being cheated on and his jealousy of professional men desiring me because of my skirt, fed my fear of being beautiful. He was emotionally triggered, and he couldn't control his rudeness toward me. I was ashamed to have a husband who rejected me.

Less than a year into my terrible, but rather educational, new marriage, I got the hint that my beauty wasn't acceptable on three separate occasions. When it came to men at work, men as friends, or the silence of the skirt. I sabotaged health with boxes of cookies per Chapter 3. My spouse's fear of abandonment created real fat on my body. I was flabbergasted with authentic flab.

His mistrust caused me to feel unsafe in my soul. My lack of soul safety translated into excess fat because of my fear of rejection and jealousy from my own husband. He had no reason to ever worry about infidelity.

But his past experiences, and to his credit, my past before marriage, made me fear my own beauty. My insecurity and fear of rejection allowed myself to eat over it. Then, I wondered, *Would he leave me? Does he love me? Am I good enough for him?*

For Tamara, jealousy came from her closest family members.

"Oh, now you're a size six and think you're so hot?" Her sister said, shoving the purple dress in Tamara's fitting room.

"Thanks," Tamara said. Jackie, her sister, didn't seem to treat her in the same loving way since she lost seventy pounds over the past year.

Their favorite pastime of going shopping seemed like a chore now—a chore of keeping up with her sister's teasing comments. Jealousy saturated Jackie's presence.

"I feel so good. It's great to wear clothes that feel good on me," Tamara said, turning around, happy with the dress and her shape in the three-way mirror. "How do I look?"

"It's alright," Jackie replied, as she rolled her eyes and landed them in the stink eye position.

This didn't only happen when shopping but also at family dinners and in conversations. Tamara knew her sister talked about her to other family members when she wasn't around. She suspected Jackie's jealousy because her sister was always the *thin one* before Tamara lost the weight. Over the next several months, tension grew in the relationship, and Tamara went back to her chubby choices because unconsciously she didn't want to continue to hurt Jackie's feelings.

Tamara wrestled with thoughts like, *I can't seem to make her happy. Is my weight making her so jealous that it'll change our relationship? Will she keep distancing herself from me if I stay in this slim body? We're so close, who else would I confide in?*

Probable Causes of the Fear of Loss or Abandonment

- We're in a relationship with someone who is jealous or controlling about how we look.
- We are in an emotionally abusive relationship.
- We haven't developed boundaries.
- We have a poor sense of self.
- We are in a codependent relationship that doesn't allow us to be a unique, empowered individual.

Reflection Question: Have you resolved your fear of loss?

Jealousy and insecurity from people we love can make us scared of losing them and our relationships, so we put the chubby suits back on to keep us and them safe from this loss. The problem is an insecure spouse can cause trouble for your waistline because they fear losing you to your new possibilities that come with your new trim self.

Jealousy shows up when you're teased, emotionally shut out, accused of cheating and flirting, or other attacks on your character based on your newfound confidence and attractiveness.

I've witnessed some cases where a spouse may fatten their spouse up so other intimate issues are avoided, such as sexual relations. Or to prevent their spouse from being as attractive to other people.

Your loved one's jealousy or insecurity carries an unspoken current as if to say, *If the weight goes, I go.* The weight can be the result of serious marital tensions that need professional as well as pastoral counseling support.

To be clear, please don't divorce your insecure partner! Many underlying tensions can be cleared up as you develop identity security in your whole self. Your spouse's insecurities or jealousies don't have to affect how you treat yourself. If they're not okay, you can still be okay. We are to bear one another's burdens in a sense of prayer and support, not bear their burdens for them to become harmful to us.

In codependent relationships one partner is considered the problem and the other partner acts as the savior. This is unhealthy because for a relationship to be done well, we need to have strong boundaries about who we are in place, so we don't get lost in someone else and take their fears and insecurities out on ourselves.

Be willing to let go of your own fear of their insecurities or jealousies. For Tamara, she learned how to acknowledge the jealousy by directly talking to her sister heart-to-heart. She shared how Jackie's actions affected her.

Tamara encouraged her sister's desire to lose weight. Jealousy is wanting something someone else has but not knowing how to attain it for yourself. Tamara didn't have to make her sister's jealousy her issue and sabotage herself over it.

Don't play small so someone else can feel big. Gain more confidence in your healthy and fit you. Stand in who you are regardless of negativity from others. As you stand firm in your identity, own your stuff and let them own theirs. As we gain a true sense of self, instead of buying other people's insecurities, we can happily return them back to the sender. Your insecurity package was delivered to the wrong person!

If this is a big struggle for you, a fantastic way to honor someone is to pray for them (alone or with them) about their insecurities.

Also do some work on your personal boundaries, as speaker Barbra Russell says in her mighty little book, *Yes! I said No!* "People pleasing is not a spiritual gift."[9] Books, such as Barbra's for a quick read or *Boundaries* by Drs. Henry Cloud and John Townsend for more depth, are sure to help you create better boundaries to strengthen how you want to be in a relationship with yourself and others despite their insecurities.

> " Stand in who you are regardless of negativity from others. "

The way I've set boundaries is a four-step process.

First, I figure out what I want. I don't want to feel ignored when I look good.

Second, I find a consequence if the person doesn't honor it. When he does that to me, I will insist on meeting with a counselor.

Third, I share my boundary and consequence with the person. "I don't want to feel ignored when I look good, so if that happens again, I'll insist on meeting with a counselor."

Fourth, I do what I say I am going to do if that happens again.

Boundary creation doesn't have to be hard, it just has to be done to manage your own peace well.

Threat #7 – Deep Life Disappointments
Chubbological Trigger – Dealing with Emotional Pain

Peggy, an independent business owner, had undergone significant financial hardships. In a session, Peggy realized that the root of her weight was her failing her own expectations. The weight served as a type of excuse.

She thought, *As long as I'm overweight, I can blame my lack of success on it.*

Irrational to say the least, but it was true for her. When she lost weight and couldn't meet her expectations that a trimmer body was supposed to give her—financial business success, she regained it. She gained and lost weight four times over the past two decades. Each time she lost, she understood she'd sabotaged her healthy habits due to using her weight as an excuse.

Her chubby suit served as the reason why she'd been financially unsuccessful in business. If she became her whole self, she would have to be more financially successful.

Not six figures, but seven figures. This unrealistic goal gave her a hidden figure. Her unrealistic expectations of herself stemmed from unresolved unforgiveness. Peggy had to deal with her reality of not being as successful as she had wanted to be at her age and her poor relationship with money; otherwise, she'd stay stuck in her overweight excuse, keeping her broke and big.

Unconsciously she thought, *If I let go of my weight, I'll have to prove myself in other areas. What if I'm a complete failure in life?*

Probable Causes of the Fear of Dealing with Emotional Pain

- We're misaligned with our soul's heart and purpose.
- We're refusing to deal with life's failures, disappointments, and griefs.
- We're misaligned with God's will for our lives.
- We're not learning the lessons life is trying to teach us.
- We have a poor relationship with life.

Reflection Question: Have you come to terms with where you are or what you have been through in life?

We cause and create our weight problem to avoid other problems.

> One of the most productive things we can do as eaters, foodies, and Chubby Church members is feel.

We cause and create our weight problem to avoid other problems. Our weight can be a mask over emotional pain that needs to be addressed. If we use our weight, like Peggy, as an excuse for why we're not as successful as we think we should be, and we lose the weight and are still not as successful as we think we should be, we must face realities of emotional pain that we've avoided with weight drama or we'll create weight drama again to avoid emotional pain.

Fear of emotional pain can accompany previously mentioned threats. Weight can be regained to avoid the emotional pain of dealing with a marriage riddled with years of tension or disagreement or past deaths of loved ones that aren't fully grieved, like my father's loss, or things we feel we should've had but didn't, like a loving parent, child, or spouse.

Perhaps we've had some trouble in life such as drug, alcohol, debt, gambling, or pornography addictions, and we have avoided dealing with the emotional pain of the losses of years, relationships, dignity, or material items our affliction has cost us. One of the most productive things we can do as eaters, foodies, is feel.

Feeling is hard because of our dysfunctional past telling us not to feel.

And life can be hard.

We may be seriously disappointed that things didn't work out as planned or expected. We may have to grieve not only the loss or hardship, but also going through the loss and hardship itself. Feeling is the key.

We'll learn how to process these threats and feel as we enact an Emotional Strength Training Plan in the Emotional Fitness Workout™ in Chapter 18. But know God is with you and wants to take your emotional burden from you. Will you give your emotional pain to your healer?

Master Your Chubbology

There you have it. Seven psychological reasons we've been super scared to drop the weight. I've officially got "all up in your business," as they'd say in Jersey. Why? Because if we don't deal with this real stuff, we'll keep stuffing.

> " Master your chubbology to break the cycle of using weight to self-protect. "

Master your chubbology to break the cycle of using weight to self-protect. And while knowing this insight is good, we need to do something about it. A good therapist can help you to heal them.

We can't and don't need to address everything at once. Just breathe. And pray through any sense of being overwhelmed. Ask the Holy Spirit, "Which of the seven threats should I address right now?" Pick one.

Answer the reflection question of the chubbological threat you sense you're going to focus on right now in your notebook. The same one you're logging observations on Inner Glutton and Diet Nut.

Do your best to pray through the stirring in your heart. Pour out your heart on paper so you're less likely to eat over what's eating you about your chubbology.

Each threat represents excess weight on the body. These and other threats resolve the more we resolve who we are.

May God's shield of protection fill your soul with safety and security quickly.

REFLECT & SHARE

1. Which chubbological threat resonated with you the most?

_____

_____

_____

_____

_____

2. What do you need to believe about the world to feel more safe in your soul?

_____

_____

_____

_____

_____

3. What boundaries will you need to be successful to let go of excess weight?

_____

_____

_____

_____

_____

CHAPTER 17

ADOPT THE FREEDOM MINDSET

Chain #2 - The Dieter's Mindset

Our minds are like a dog without a leash.

Diet Nut, the alter ego of Inner Glutton, creates the dieter's mindset. Diets are the American way. It's estimated that 45 million Americans diet regularly and participate in a $66 billion dollar industry.[1] About 97 million Americans try a new fad diet every year.[2] John LaRose, research director of Market Data Enterprise, said, "America's dieters are fickle and shift from fad to fad."[3]

Someone is profiting on diets, why isn't it you?

We've believed lies for too long. Reduce the assault on your results by adopting a freedom mindset and quit being duped into temporary gimmicks.

Chains keep us stuck in bondage. The chain we need to destroy in this chapter is our dieter's mindset.

A mindset is a collection of thoughts that over a period of time influences the way we perceive life. You have a collection of individual thoughts and experiences that over the course of your life has accumulated in your head when it comes to diets, weight, body image, food, and eating. This library of thoughts and images has formed your mindset.

To find out how affected you are by the dieter's mindset, let me ask you a few questions.

DIETER'S MINDSET STRONGHOLD QUIZ

Put a check next to the answer that describes your mindset and add the total points below. The higher the score, the more the dieter's mindset is in motion.

1. How often do you speak or think harshly about your body?
☐(5) ALWAYS ☐(4) OFTEN ☐(3) SOMETIMES ☐(2) RARELY ☐(1) NEVER

- -

2. How often do you eat without discretion because you've messed up your diet anyway?
☐(5) ALWAYS ☐(4) OFTEN ☐(3) SOMETIMES ☐(2) RARELY ☐(1) NEVER

- -

3. How often do you search for a new diet?
☐(5) ALWAYS ☐(4) OFTEN ☐(3) SOMETIMES ☐(2) RARELY ☐(1) NEVER

- -

4. How often do you attempt to diet?
☐(5) ALWAYS ☐(4) OFTEN ☐(3) SOMETIMES ☐(2) RARELY ☐(1) NEVER

- -

5. How often do you feel guilty or like you've "cheated" when you've eaten what you enjoy?
☐(5) ALWAYS ☐(4) OFTEN ☐(3) SOMETIMES ☐(2) RARELY ☐(1) NEVER

- -

6. How often do you worry about or count grams or calories?
☐(5) ALWAYS ☐(4) OFTEN ☐(3) SOMETIMES ☐(2) RARELY ☐(1) NEVER

- -

7. How often is your motive for exercise to lose weight?
☐(5) ALWAYS ☐(4) OFTEN ☐(3) SOMETIMES ☐(2) RARELY ☐(1) NEVER

- -

8. How often do you eliminate whole food groups because you're on a diet?
☐(5) ALWAYS ☐(4) OFTEN ☐(3) SOMETIMES ☐(2) RARELY ☐(1) NEVER

- -

9. How often do you eat something you think is "bad"?
☐(5) ALWAYS ☐(4) OFTEN ☐(3) SOMETIMES ☐(2) RARELY ☐(1) NEVER

- -

10. How often does the number on the scale dictate your mood for the day?
☐(5) ALWAYS ☐(4) OFTEN ☐(3) SOMETIMES ☐(2) RARELY ☐(1) NEVER

- -

Total Score:

Score Sheet
30–50 | Free your mind and the rest will follow!
20–30 | You've done some mindset work and it shows!
10–20 | You're freeing your mind to the next level!

_____

Adopt the Weight & Eating Freedom Mindset

A healthy mindset will set you emotionally and mentally free from the destructive thoughts that drive weight and eating obsession.

Our results in life manifest *creative inputs,* such as thoughts, emotions, beliefs, and actions. Thoughts both shape and create reality. Think of them as seeds. The mind is fertile ground cultivated by thought seeds. And these seeds can be beneficial or harmful.

Your mind has no judgment around the thoughts. As a fertile ground it grows them with the water of your own behavior, emotions, and beliefs. So, your thoughts yield a crop you can see in your reality—one you like or one you'd rather feed to the birds.

The tree of our thought life produces fruit. For our reality to change, we need to have a change of mind and heart.

Figure 17.1 Your Manifested Reality

Good news, Dr. Caroline Leaf, a neurobiology researcher, in her book *Who Switched Off My Brain,* confirmed it's possible to reframe the brain by taming the thoughts in your mind in what science calls neuroplasticity.[4]

Albert Einstein said, "We can't change a problem with the same thinking used to create it."[5]

Can you see how the wrong mindset is a chain that keeps us going in circles in the soul wilderness? A freedom mindset begins with strengthening your mental fitness. Yes, there's a workout for everything.

The Mental Fitness Workout

We're going to eliminate this mental chub by practicing mental fitness. Let's be like Wonder Woman or John Wayne and lasso bondage thoughts. We're going to snatch them up, bring them close to our eyes, and examine the fruit of our reality that our thoughts create and implant new thought seeds and actions.

This workout is hard in the sense that you have an estimated 48.6 thoughts per minute, or up to 70,000 thoughts per day.[6] But easy, because it's only three steps.

First, you identify negative/unhealthy thoughts related to food, dieting, weight, and eating, such as: *I can't eat carbs, I've got to start my diet on Monday,* or *I think this new workout plan will help me lose thirty pounds this month.* Thoughts like these will enter the lasso.

Second, you exchange those thoughts with freedom beliefs like: *I choose not to eat foods that don't provide nutritional value, I live healthy now,* or *Not so fast get-skinny-quick-scheme, I'm onto you and it's one day at a time!*

As a third step, question the thought and the belief it stands on. From now on don't let a thought go by without a question. Ask yourself: *Is this true? What fruit is this producing?* or *Is this helping or hurting me?* Deeper beliefs under the thoughts are usually some variation of I'm not healthy enough, skinny enough, good enough, fit enough, acceptable enough, loveable enough—yada, yada, yada. If we repeat a lie enough times, we accept it as truth.

Once you own these new beliefs, you create a new mindset. But the next step is not only a freedom mindset but also freedom action, which is something you'll do differently going forward. Freedom actions create a powerful punch through the walls of bondage. You'll carry out a freedom action to support your new freedom mindset.

Adopt the Freedom Mindset

Let's expose seven unhealthy mindsets that need to be eliminated from our thinking and the corresponding freedom mindset and freedom actions to slim down mental chub.

Belief #1 – There's a Magic Pill

"There's got to be a solution that makes me lose weight fast."

Shelley couldn't zip her favorite pair of jeans, so she raced to Walmart and filled her cart with protein powders, diet pills, and a bottle of appetite suppressants. At the checkout stand, she added to her purchases a magazine that promised, "Lose 10 pounds in 10 days!"

Last night, Shelley ate half a jar of peanut butter. Anxious, she reasons, *I can't afford to buy a cart load of new clothes to accommodate my expanding muffin top.* Shelley's upset her peanut butter binge caused her clothes not to fit that morning, but in truth, it's her quest for a magic pill to fix the damage that's ill fitting.

This scenario is common for dieters. We get deceived because dieting is based in deception. Real diets only work when there's a full lifestyle change, such as vegetarian or gluten free, an acute health issue like diabetes or high blood pressure, or for a short term affair.

A magic pill sounds so soothing, so helpful, so immediate. Think about it, isn't this a cycle that only sets us up for failure?

When we search for a get-skinny-quick scheme, don't we end up relying on that scheme rather than taking responsibility and owning our choices today? In our heroic quest, with a Diet Nut logo'd cape flapping in the wind, we point our finger to the sky, and say, "Where's the next great diet pill. Then, I will eat better!"

Why Magic Pill Hunting Doesn't Work

The get skinny quick belief robs us of *being* healthy now. We tend to postpone good eating habit until later, and engage in poor eating now, because of the hope a magic pill is coming.

The magic pill is knowing there's no such thing as a magic pill because it doesn't exist. The real magic pill is to reject the fantasy of a magic pill and embrace the certainty of the daily body habits, twenty four hours of grace, one day a time. If we don't have a magic pill to pretend to find and struggle to stick to, we can take responsibility for our health today.

When you get duped by the latest diet fad, you make a choice to avoid a true commitment to a lifetime commitment of healthy eating because you're going for the quick fix. True health is a lifelong process. Dieting is a distraction from true health.

Some people set weight loss time frames like they would for other tasks, such as cleaning the garage or finishing a project. It doesn't work well like this for us. What happens if you start a diet plan, believing that in three months you'll lose fifty pounds? You'll eat as though you can lose the weight in days, not daily efforts.

I know because I popped diet pills, tried dozens of diets, and bought all the *National Enquirer* headlined papers that promised me fast weight loss.

A magic pill, the quest for a get-skinny-quick plan, pill, or program distracts from your real success of one day at time healthy habits to create a lifetime of healthy eating.

Freedom Mindset – "I live healthy now"

Ending the dieter's mindset will require you to live a twenty four hour day and get on track immediately, as opposed to waiting to start eating healthy tomorrow or when you find the next *lose weight fast* plan. This also includes not starting your repair diet on Monday or any other day of the week. Why Monday? Forty six percent of diets start on Mondays.[7]

To live healthy now means that no matter what day it is, no matter where you are, and no matter what foods are available or not available, you can still choose wisely that day.

You'll eliminate the holiday or vacation syndrome—when you eat like you're a linebacker trying to make the college team just because it's a holiday or because you're on vacation. Transition your mindset to live healthy now. Allow for one day at a time, a twenty four hour day of grace, moment by moment, choice by choice. Drop the fantasy. It's consistent changes over time that create lasting results.

Freedom Action – Magically Meal Plan

Make a commitment to stop magic pill hunting. Instead, meal plan to reduce the intensive impulse to jump on another diet bandwagon. Meal planning is proven to support healthier eating and healthier families. In one study, researchers found that families who sit down and eat together are less likely to be obese.[8]

For us not to worry about Inner Glutton derailing the day and triggering Diet Nut, we need to consider an intentional meal plan.

How to Magically Meal Plan

1. Set your intention on what you'll eat the next day, the night before. Jot down what you intend to eat on a post-it note. If you're wondering what to eat for dinner, you've already lost, and Inner Glutton is more vulnerable to acting out.

2. Decide when to meal plan. Figure out what habit is easier for you to stick with—the night before, at the start of the week, or every two to three days. I prefer the night before, but early on in my journey,

I would plan the whole week's meals. It also helps to create a master list of meals. You can make a list on paper, on index cards, with a meal planning app, or on your computer. A list of about five to ten meal ideas for breakfast, lunch, and dinner works.

3. Decide when to grocery shop. Grocery shopping is a nemesis for those who suffer from weight and eating issues. We tend to eat out or neglect our eating, which makes us vulnerable to our Inner Glutton taking over.

    Consider the same day of the week to grocery shop. Lonna reduces the time it takes to grocery shop with an app. She shops on the app, then picks up her groceries at a scheduled time or has them delivered.

Belief #2 – The Drive to Lose Weight
"I've got to lose weight."

I'd been diligent—hired a personal trainer and made five trips to the gym each week. Fifteen rounds of strength building and a boatload of kickbox cardio later, I excitedly anticipated what the scale would show that morning at weigh-in as I walked into the gym.

I stood on the scale wearing a new brown skirt and a lightweight cream jacket that wouldn't add extra ounces. Marilyn, my personal trainer, edged the slide on the scale carefully before she announced the result.

"One hundred ninety pounds," she said in a matter of fact tone.

Then something welled up so fast inside of me I didn't dare try to control it … then it hit.

"Baawaaaaah," an inconsolable tear dam broke, at the gym, in front of innocent, muscular gym rats—unbeknownst to me or them what was happening.

"Why won't it move?" I kicked the scale as I wiped off the mascara trickling down my face.

I worked out with a personal trainer and ate zero calorie products for crying out loud. *Why didn't the scale reflect my efforts? And why was I crying profusely in public?!* I thought hurrying out.

All I thought about was weight loss. I exercised to lose weight, ate to lose weight, but I never seemed to lose much weight.

Out of frustration, I ditched Marilyn and the local health club. Defeated, I spent the next few months paving my way to heart attack city with continual stops at the local Wendy's for a sausage, egg, and cheese biscuit, binge visits for drug store candy, and lonely depressed nights talking to random, way underqualified friend therapists on the phone for hours. Yet my mind still dwelled on losing weight.

I developed a pattern of yo-yo exercise. You know how you exercise one week and then you're off for the next year? I enthusiastically started only to stop again. Why did I do this? Why couldn't I sustain an exercise program? Or an eating program?

Because the only benefit I truly cared about when it came to exercise or eating was weight loss, not better health, productivity, joyful emotions, or world peace—nope, just weight loss for me, my vain self, and I. If weight loss didn't come fast enough, then the exercise and the meal planning was over.

Why the Drive to Lose Weight Doesn't Work

It may be a part of your reality. You may feel you do, indisputably, need to lose weight. The doctor could've told you or your tight jeans (the ones where the button popped off at dinner a few months back). But how long have you thought about losing weight? Is the weight gone yet?

Perhaps, like a driver's manual stick shift, the very thought of losing weight is causing you to stay stuck in "losing weight" gear, never actually shifting to "lost the weight." Mind games are tricky because while it seems like common sense, this thinking doesn't work. Like I said earlier, your mind is fertile ground in which the thought seed will grow.

You tell your mind "lose weight," it takes it presently, losing weight. Your mind only knows what's right now. The difference in thinking is the difference between having to lose the weight and having lost the weight. It thinks, *lose weight, lose weight, lose weight*, so you have a present condition of weight to lose. Make sense?

Freedom Mindset – "I am healthy"

What do healthy people do? We want the results of healthy people, and we know what to do, but we don't believe we're healthy. Dieters don't believe they're healthy, which means the actions of healthy activities are short lived.

Our beliefs impact our actions, and our actions impact our results. We don't need to lose weight, we need to *be* healthy. And we need *to believe* we are healthy now to start doing healthy things. People who think they need to lose weight don't believe they're healthy and deceive themselves into another diet.

We're called human beings for a reason. We operate best in the principle of be-do-have versus the other way around. We control by forcing our next diet, attempting to work out for hours or drink gallons of water per day, which is human doing. We body manipulate to force the body to endure our short lived dieting tactics.

The principle be-do-have suggests that out of who we believe we are is what we do. Out of what we do is what we have or the results we get. Being is the essence of our beliefs that underlie our actions.

When we concentrate on being healthy, we tend to become healthier and make better choices. When we believe we're healthy and fit, we'll do healthy and fit things and ultimately have a healthy and less flabby body.

Funny, not in a humorous way, but in an ironic way, the drive to lose weight puts us in a state of being—well, fat.

Freedom Action — Live Like You're Already Your Desired Size

What if you were already the size you wanted to be? How would you be any different? What would you do differently than you may be doing now? Wouldn't those actions lead you to the health you wanted to have? It's a good practice to live as though you're maintaining the weight you've wanted to lose.

Instead of the idea of losing weight, we're going to be and act as though the weight is already lost. What got you to a size 14 won't get you to a size 10. We'll deal with the battles of overeating and food addiction in Book 2, but think about how you've lived in the someday maybe space with your health.

We think because we know we need to lose weight, and weight is driving our thoughts, that we can just lose it later. Yet, later doesn't come, and weight gain is still a reality. Our actions must be based on living at our desired place today.

How to Live Like You're Already Your Desired Size

1. Talk to people at your desired size. Ask what they do to stay healthy. Chances are you could write a book on health material with all the diets you've done over the years. But take some time to find someone at work, Facebook, work, or the local health club whom you admire and pick his or her brain a bit for deeper insights.

2. Do those things. Focus on your vision from the action chapter and practice being at your desired size, no matter what things look like today.

3. Finish this book, take the Whole & Free Health online program, and get the T-shirt. Find out more at *www.thechubbychurch.com*.

Belief #3 – Cheating on Diet with Foods

"I've been good all week so I can cheat just this once."

Ken, a middle aged salesman, loved his quarter pounder with cheese. His demanding job required a lot of road time and fast food provided convenient meals. But Ken hated the belly fat his chubby choices produced, so when he could barely button his pants, he'd ignite his get-skinny-quick diet plan.

And the first thing to go? You guessed it, his quarter pounder with cheese. He knew this supersized meal wasn't beneficial, so he cut it out. As usual, it worked for a few days, but one particularly stressful day at work, he found himself at the drive through window. He told his wife when he got home, guilt ridden, "I cheated." He referred not to her, but to his diet.

Why Cheating with Food Doesn't Work

Cheat. It's not an endearing word, is it? Cheat stirs up dark emotions of shame and deception. The problem with cheating on your own decision to eat well, is an all or nothing definition of the word healthy. As a result, we swing from dieting one day to cheating and possibly to out-of-control the next.

You've tried to rationalize popular diet advice to have a cheat day, but after the so-called cheat day, you still have tormenting guilt and take several days to get back on track from overindulgence.

Not only does cheating on a diet cause you to feel guilty, it also causes you to eat well for a temporary period and disregards your favorite fun foods in a delusional forever fear frenzy. Ultimately you cheat yourself out of mental freedom. This on-again, off-again relationship with healthy eating and living must come to an end.

Freedom Mindset – "I'm in a monogamous relationship with healthy eating and living"

A healthy lifestyle includes having food for pleasure, as well as for nutrition. There's no need to continue to "cheat" or be "off" of your eating. Divorce the concept of diets and explore a new world of options for a true healthy lifestyle. Healthy living is a lifestyle that includes some of the foods you currently reject when you diet.

For example, if you believe having a cupcake is cheating, you're now on a diet, setting yourself up for guilt and failure when you have a cupcake. However, if your mindset shifts to living in a monogamous relationship with health, you can expand your definition of health to include a cupcake occasionally.

Would it be possible to eliminate the word *cheat* from your vocabulary when it comes to diet? And expand your definition of health to include your favorites?

Freedom Action – Expand Your Definition of Health

By expanding your definition of health, you can increase foods that are positively impacting your health and decrease foods negatively impacting nutritional health. Imagine your best foods hit a bullseye. Bullseye foods keep you on track to feel your best energy and confidence.

Occasionally you'll hit outside of the bullseye, hence Ken's quarter pounder. True healthy living includes foods you enjoy. It's the frequency, quality, timing, and size of that choice that changes.

How to Expand Your Definition of Health So You Don't Have to Cheat on Your Healthy Life

Figure 17.2 Inclusive Healthy Eating

In the next belief we'll discuss the meaning of the three new food groups. But to expand your definition, you can look at what you eat most of the time and include your favorites on occasion. Make your own chart like above and include the foods that meet the descriptions below.

1. The bullseye at the center includes the foods that make you feel great, the ones you consider healthy. They provide your body with value. Eat these foods most of the time.

2. The middle circle includes foods that make you feel good, you consider them healthy, but you need to be mindful of how much of them you eat.

3. The outer circle includes the food and drinks that make you feel like a cheat. But you include a cheat food, as a treat, at a lesser frequency, better quality, or reduced caloric load. For example, a cookie from refined flour to a whole grain alternative version.

The dieter's mindset can make one cupcake turn into five cupcakes in a nanosecond. In the freedom mindset you can eat a cupcake and have peace about it because you're no longer a slave to the cupcake nor cheating on your diet when you eat one.

The guilt dissipates and now you can bask in the wonderful feeling of food freedom. To sum it up, expand your definition of health to include healthy alternatives of your favorites.

Belief #4 – Food has Morals

"Brownies are so bad."

I once watched a group of women and a group of teenage boys in the same environment, at a friend's Bible study. Without being too weird, I was looking at how they approached eating these little cookies.

The women were selective, only eating one or two. The young men could care less, and they on average ate about five to seven. This was interesting to me because the comments of the women were, "I can't eat too many cookies," or "I don't want to eat like a pig," or "I need to lose weight so I shouldn't be eating these."

Those cookies were plagued by guilt.

The young guys were just thinking, *These cookies look good, so I'll eat some.* They kept it simple, no stories around it, and most certainly no guilt. There's nothing wrong with eating five to seven cookies. What's crazy for us is to eat five to seven cookies with the expectation of losing weight or only having one or two cookies because we're scared to death to gain weight. This isn't freedom.

Why Assigning Moral Value to Food Doesn't Work

Food doesn't have moral value. It's like money. You've heard it said that the love of money is the root of all evil. Is the money evil? No, the people who love money more than what's right are evil. People are the ones who have been divinely made to have moral consciousness and who can operate in good or bad ways. From now on, let go of the thought that any particular food is bad or good.

Freedom Mindset – "There's no such thing as morally good or bad food!"

What happens when you think the chocolate bar is bad? Psychologically, you're validating shame and telling yourself that you're bad because you want something "bad." The cookie is an innocent bystander in the shame and guilt sandwich. When you eat it, you feel bad about yourself!

Deep down inside it comes with feelings of guilt, which is feeling bad! Logically, I'm sure you prefer to feel good. So, why not call food what it is—a chocolate bar that you enjoyed. When you eat "bad" you feel badly that you ate badly, and the demoralization continues to create the same poor eating behaviors.

Humans do have moral consciences; therefore, we can project our deep feelings of shame onto others and inanimate objects like food. There's no such thing as a morally good or bad food. There are beneficial and non-beneficial choices for your body, but food itself is neutral.

> **The cookie is an innocent bystander in the shame and guilt sandwich.**

Freedom Action – Neutralize Food

An Alternative Way to Think about Food

There are three categories of food that we eat:

Nutritious. (N) Nutritious foods have the ability to heal and restore your body's balance. While these foods may not always be the best tasting (Brussel sprouts or liver, for example), —they give your body what it needs to thrive.

Nutritious & Delicious. (ND) Nutritious and delicious foods are foods that feel good to eat and you enjoy the taste. My favorites are mangos, cherries, or a kale salad with salmon. These are flavors you enjoy and that pack a powerful nutritional punch.

Delicious. (D) Delicious foods have virtually no nutritional value, but they make your taste buds dance a jig! While, these foods can be explicit, appealing to your carnal lust nature, it's unrealistic to cut them out completely.

As discussed in the body section, most food is loaded with high fructose corn syrup, sodium, and fat to addict your brain. You can't blame your taste buds for wanting all that manipulated flavor. Nutritious and nutritious & delicious foods won't create a sense of strong craving. You can enjoy them and enjoy the full freedom of your own mind—a mind that isn't captured by your food and weight thoughts.

It's okay to enjoy delicious foods, like cupcakes, cake, crackers, and other tongue rock stars. Just eat them with a frequency that allows you to stay free from food and weight drama. And change from refined versions to better quality. We'll discuss how to eat your delectables in Book 2.

What's great about just calling the food delicious versus bad is that it reflects positively on your self-esteem and your emotions. When you eat delicious food, enjoy it with a smile and savor each bite. It'll feel energetically positive in your soul. You feel good about the delicious choices you made. When you're eating delicious foods, the key is to watch the frequency, quality, timing, and size.

While I am a big advocate for dramatically reducing sugar and refined flour goods due to their negative effects on the brain and body, I think it's unrealistic to expect yourself to never eat delicious foods. Food is for celebration, too. It's meant to be enjoyed.

But per our body habits conversations, if we're a slave to pleasure or only delicious manmade foods, we'll reap great problems in our health.

Are you ready to enjoy your food and take off the good and bad labels?

> " When you eat delicious food, enjoy it with a smile and savor each bite. "

Belief #5 – Worth as Thinness

"I am worthy of love when I'm thin."

"Listen, you're beautiful and everything, but you need to lose ten pounds for me to be with you," said a man to a woman.

Click, tat, click, tat. The sound of that women's heels walking away.

Conditional love is not love. If anyone treated us as poorly as we can treat ourselves in the weight and worth area, most of us would leave.

Ty, a beautiful young African American woman wanted to be married.

"What's stopping you," I asked.

"My weight! I don't want to attract a guy like this."

"Why not?" I asked.

"Because, Jendayi, I just don't feel like anyone would really love me like this. I feel like any guy would really want there to be less of me to love, you know," she said, laughing nervously.

"So, you want someone who loves you because you're a certain size?" I asked.

Ty furrowed her brow and said, "Well, no, I want someone to love me for me."

"Hmm, does that sound like conditional or unconditional love?" I asked. "Ty, you're beautiful on the outside, and you're shining on the inside. When you get love based on what you look like, you'll fight for unconditional love in the relationship by gaining weight. You've experienced conditional love in the past. It was based on how you looked and how you performed. Is that the love you want for your future?"

Open her eyes.

"No," she replied. She had humbly received the truth that she was worthy of love now, not after she got skinny enough to receive it. The revelation was touching to her as she tried on the new truth.

Rena was told that it was her weight that made a guy she liked run away. Thankfully, one day when discussing her love life with a friend, Rena admitted she felt she should lose weight so the right guy would come along.

Her loving friend said, "What if you found a man that accepted you as you are and loved who you are, exactly as you are?"

This revelation stirred deep tears from Rena. She accepted herself instead of believing she needed to be anything different to attract her spouse. She's been married for about a decade to her husband who met her at her heaviest weight. He loved her for both who and how she was.

> " Your body shape and size have nothing to do with your true worth. "

Why Worth in Thinness Doesn't Work

You don't have to be skinny to be approved, loved, valued, worthy, beautiful, or powerful. The truth is you're all of these things right now. Your body shape and size have nothing to do with your true worth.

Remain open, whoever you choose to be with will love you for your spirit and soul expressed through your body. However, how you eat and feel about yourself determines how much worth you feel inside. Eat like you love yourself.

Freedom Mindset – "I'm worthy of love because I'm loved by God!"

We're not to live defeated, worthless, and devalued. When you buy a new television, you want to utilize it for its purpose, right?

You are good enough. You have purpose.

You are loved for simply being a human being.

Somewhere down the line you've learned that flaws, wrinkles, and wobbly arms aren't deserving of love, so you place your worth in being better looking.

Please accept that you are perfectly imperfect.

Freedom Action – Place Your Worth God's Love

Where do you place your worth? Imagine your soul being like a ball. Your name is on that ball. It's a gorgeous ball, made of gold and silver with rare gems, like pearls or diamonds.

Imagine yourself placing that precious, unique, valuable ball in a bucket that has different labels on the outside of it—labels such as education, ministry title, race, marital status, income, savings, health, weight, or talents.

When we don't feel a genuine sense of worth in who God created us to be, we will look outside of ourselves to the various labels that define worth in our view.

One of my worth buckets was labeled "skinny." Earlier attempts at weight loss caused me to have fleeting self-worth. When skinny, I felt superior, but when chubby, I felt inferior. Inferiority/superiority complexes happen when our worth is unstable. If we're pleased with our bucket label of weight, education, income, marital status, or health, it can bring out a superior, arrogant, puffed up, conceited, self-absorbed, and trite side of us.

If we are displeased with our weight and other bucket labels, it can bring out an inferior, depressed, deflated, defeated, isolated, and neglectful side. Yet, both fruits of arrogance and depression have the same root in chronically low self-worth or lack of self-value.

> "Inferiority/superiority complexes happen when our worth is unstable."

Where have you placed your soul's worth?

How to Place Your Worth

1. Speak to the label that's been stealing your worth. For example - You can take your self-worth out of the scale by speaking to it. Speak to the scale and tell it who's boss. It sounds something like this, "Scale, you are not going to predict my mood any longer. I am enough! I am more than what I weigh."

2. Keep growing your identity in truth.

Belief #6 – Thinness Equates to Happiness
"I can't be happy, until I lose weight."

Danielle participated in a healing retreat I lead called *The Hungry Soul*. During our discussion time, as I led a teaching on the interrelationship between body, soul, and spirit, Danielle revealed her true belief: if she was overweight, she was destined to be unhappy.

She insisted and almost yelled at me.

"Jendayi, how in the world can I be happy being seventy five pounds overweight?! You can't be happy and fat!" her voice echoed in the large great room of my Denver condo.

We sat at the dining room table as I taught on giant post-it notes on the wall of our intimate retreat.

"What's bigger, Danielle, your soul, which is who you are, or your body?" I replied. We don't get who we are, so we're often limited by the sight of our bodies.

Danielle studied the flipchart at the front of the room that contained a diagram of interlocking circles to represent body, soul, and spirit as she pondered my comment. She looked that diagram up and down several times. Tears clouded her eyes.

"Isn't the body an instrument for my soul?" she asked.

"So, which is bigger?" I repeated.

"My soul?" she asked.

"So, where does happiness come from?" I asked.

"My soul?" she asked again.

"Danielle, who makes you happy?" I asked, driving the lesson home.

"I do," Danielle said as her frown turned into a smile, revealing her newfound understanding.

Why Waiting to Lose Weight to Be Happy Doesn't Work

Waiting to lose weight to be happy puts your life on hold. In exchange for an adventurous life out and about in God's beautiful creation, you're stuck watching television, watching YouTube videos, watching everyone's wall on Facebook, and watching your own life go by.

And while you're watching, waiting to be slim so you can be happy, you've got to have your popcorn, right?

Don't postpone living any longer. Weight isn't your problem. Your discontentment is. Unhappy people are people who don't know who they are or whose they are yet.

You put off doing fun things, meeting new people, and doing what you've always wanted. We're suspended on hold until this weight problem goes away. The problem is that it never seems to go away—for good anyway.

> "Weight isn't your problem. Your discontentment is."

A lack of contentment in body produces an unsafe feeling in the soul, and an unsafe soul—that isn't feeling good enough to be happy now—will create a self-protection barrier in weight on the body. Oh, and more than 43 percent of people with depression are obese.[9] And 38 percent of obese people are depressed.[10] It's time to think and do something differently.

Freedom Mindset – "I choose to be happy in my size now!"

Marci Shimoff, author of *Happy for No Reason: 7 Steps to Being Happy from the Inside Out*, said, "To become happier we have to snap out of the trance that our happiness rests in 'more and better' which we'll get 'someday.' No matter what we have, *Happy for No Reason* exists only now, not later."[11]

Create a life you enjoy and love, just put the weight thing on the back burner, and put loving yourself and being content with who you are on the front burner. Better soul care leads to a healthier, happier body.

Your soul has been oppressed because of the whole weight and eating thing. It wants to come out and play. Make happiness a choice in your current size to produce soul safety to let the weight go as you embrace more of you—and more of life.

When you're unhappy at your current weight with unresolved roots, it's only a matter of time before you'd be unhappy at a new weight. With weight and eating obsession, if we're unhappy, we eat! So eventually the same problem will happen again.

Happiness is a choice.

Joy is a fruit of your spiritual transformation.

We can be content in all circumstances when our joy comes from the inside out. Life is guaranteed to have problems, but, happiness is a choice to honor all that life has given you.

You deserve to enjoy your life and be free. Joy is a human right. May overflowing joy fill you!

> When you're unhappy at your current weight with unresolved roots, it's only a matter of time before you'd be unhappy at a new weight.

Freedom Action – Celebrate and Enjoy Your Life

If there have been activities you haven't done because your weight has stopped you, it's time to do them. Begin to live your life fully, despite your current weight condition. As you cultivate happiness in soul and joy in spirit, you'll see weight release from your body. Do this daily to create a genuine state of happiness and joy.

Choosing happiness and focusing on what's good, pure, holy, and worthy of good in your day can become your new normal. Go try a new Bible study, join a small group, go hiking, buy clothes you like, take a vacation, and wear a bathing suit. As you break free of discontent by doing what you haven't done because of weight, you'll break free.

Will you make a choice to be happy despite your body shape or life circumstances?

How to Celebrate and Enjoy Your Life

1. Make a list of all the things you'd like to do in life, then do them.

2. Cross things off the list after you complete them.

3. Meditate on all the wonderful things in your life to stir up gratitude. Gratitude creates big smiles and big joy.

Belief #7 – One Mistake Defines the Whole Day

"I messed up my eating, so I might as well eat whatever I want."

Jenna sabotaged her efforts almost daily. She'd get up with Diet Nut at her side, focusing on the perfect breakfast meal. But by lunch she couldn't resist the smell of freshly baked Danishes near her small town workplace. Jenna got her Danish and threw the rest of her healthy eating plan out the window, devouring any refined carbohydrate that crossed her path.

Candy, office birthday cake, extra mashed potatoes at dinner—nothing could escape Jenna's mouth. She thought, *I already messed up, so why bother eating well now?*

Diet Nut owned the morning, but her Inner Glutton dominated lunch through bedtime. Out of control and discouraged Jenna repeated this Groundhog Day until she changed her mindset and figured out her track.

Why One Mistake Defines the Whole Day Doesn't Work

This mindset doesn't work for obvious reasons. Health results will be delayed every time that we make a mistake and decide to wallow in it by making a dozen more the rest of the day. In the twenty four hours of grace we get each day, we'll make some mistakes, but wild eating delays our progress.

Your life isn't defined by this one area. Usually when we mess up there are other factors at work like sleep quality, things on your heart, or inadequate time with God. Think of your whole life as being on or off track so you can see when you are tracking well with God or when you're off.

Freedom Mindset – "I get back on track immediately!"

You're riding a bike down a long street and you fall off, but you still want to get home. Would you just stop riding the bike? Would you roll around on the street making your scratches worse?

It's the same case here. Dust yourself off, get back on the bike, and keep going. The bike is your commitment to freedom choices. There's no falling off the wagon in a healthy relationship with food. Be committed to your best life, no matter what bumps you hit along the road.

The sooner you get up and get back on the bike and keep riding, the more you will see the transformations take place. You can and will achieve health, but you don't throw out the whole day or night based on a mistake or two or three.

Freedom Action – Figure Out Your Track

Study yourself over the next few weeks to develop your personal on track and off track understanding. You're in the process of looking deeply at your soul, lifestyle, patterns, and environment to find out what supports you thriving.

There's a saying, "The secrets of your future are hidden in your daily routine." To find out what works best for you, start thinking about what an on track, great day looks and feels like so you can enjoy more of them.

- What does it mean to be on track in your life?
- What does it mean to be off track?
- When did you last feel great in your joy and body?
- How do you get yourself to feel good again after you've felt down?

Table 17.3 Example of Jenna's Life On and Off Track

JENNA'S LIFE ON TRACK	JENNA'S LIFE OFF TRACK
Eating according to bio-individual food plan	Eating wildly without discretion
Morning devotional completed	Skipped morning devotional
Clean house	Messy house
Exercising 4 to 6 times per week	Exercising less than 3 times per week
Planning fun activities to look forward to	Watching excessive television
Drinking water	Drinking coffee like it is water
Showing up for work on time	Late for work
Logging Inner Glutton findings as needed	Binge eating and not learning from it
Emotionally Clearing on a regular basis	Wallowing in negative emotions and thoughts
Bills are paid on time	Overspending, missing payments
Sense of contentment	Sense of overwhelm, feeling anxious or negative
Taking vitamins and supplements	Skipped vitamins and supplements
Kind toward others	Rude toward others

These questions help to describe what your life, on track, looks and feels like. We can create our lives and our outcomes.

Your life on track feels good. Really good. Words like calm, balanced, happy, fun, light, encouraging, positive, and energetic come to mind as feelings of being on track. Your life off track feels bad. Words like anxious, unbalanced, scattered, sad,

> Your life on track feels good. Really good.

dull, heavy, discouraging, negative, and drained describe being off track.

It's up to you to do the self study to find out what makes you happy and energetic. You deserve to feel great on a consistent basis.

> " It's up to you to do the self study to find out what makes you happy and energetic. "

And from this day forward, in your committed, monogamous relationship with healthy eating and living, you can refer to yourself as being on or off track. And when off track, get back on track quickly by asking the question, *What's the best thing for me to do right now?*

How to Figure Out Your Track

1. Make a two column chart. Put 'My life on track' on one side and 'My life off track' on the other side.
2. Review the questions above Table 17.3 and describe what each track looks like.
3. Going forward, refer to being on or off track and do your best to get on track quickly.

Renew Your Mind

Do you feel the heaviness lifting from your soul? The dieter's mindset is weighty. You can put the freedom mindsets on index cards or post-it notes to repeat them in your mind. We walked through the seven strongest beliefs in the dieter's mindset and exchanged them for a freedom mindset.

We've taken a break from heavy lifting in chubbology and practiced mental fitness. Coming up next is the Emotional Fitness Workout ™ to heal chubbology, as well as emotional eating.

REFLECT & SHARE

1. Which dieter's mindset belief is most difficult to release?

_____

_____

_____

_____

_____

2. Which new freedom mindset belief resonates the most?

_____

_____

_____

_____

_____

3. What new freedom action will you try?

_____

_____

_____

_____

_____

CHAPTER 18

ENACT AN EMOTIONAL STRENGTH TRAINING PLAN

Chain #3 – Emotional Eating

Out of the heart the mouth eats.

O*h, God! What did I just do?* I reached for the phone and dialed a therapist as though calling 911.

Thankfully, I got an appointment with Kali the next day.

We exchanged greetings as I entered her office. I sat on a cream colored cushioned chair. Nervous, I glanced at the wooden floors and a fireplace. The blue and cream walls matched the Denver sky. Proper degrees that hung above her desk provided me with a sense of security in her ability to help me. I exhaled a sigh of relief.

"So, what's happening with you?" she asked.

"I keep having overeating episodes," I said.

"What's that like?" she asked.

"Oh, you know, two oversized slices of pizza, a huge cinnamon roll, and a pint of butter pecan ice cream all in one sitting." Ashamed, my eyes could've burned a hole in the wooden floor.

"Why do you think you're doing this to yourself?" she asked.

"Well, I'm married, but I feel like I'm all by myself. My husband hasn't been attentive the past few months. I know he loves me, but I feel abandoned by him," I said on the brink of tears. "I keep overeating when he doesn't come home from work or prioritizes his friends over me. Do you think he's avoiding me?"

The words stung my heart as they rolled off my tongue. I felt pathetic and ashamed. I reflected on my move to Denver a year prior and tapped the iceberg of my suppressed pain of not having close friends and family around. My husband was closest to me, but it was unfair to think he could meet all my needs.

Kali proceeded to walk me through a meditation to stir up emotional memories. She asked questions to help me tap into beliefs that drove me to stuff myself.

"What's the earliest memory of feeling lonely and abandoned?" she asked in her soothing tone.

Holy Spirit, help me, I prayed.

A wellspring of grief flooded my heart as a vivid image of the scene emerged in my mind. "My father's funeral at twelve years old. He's lying in the casket and I'm looking over the casket at his sleeping face," I said.

"What do you need to say to your dad," she asked.

"I never knew you," an unconstrained shout took flight toward my dead dad, "I never knew you." I repeated several times louder and louder, as grief completely overtook my eye sockets.

Kali urged me to say all that was in my heart to say to him in my active memory movie.

This emotional baggage was completely forgotten until I confronted the matter.

My twelve-year-old self believed his death was because she was defective. His final departure created a sense of confused identity.

The revelation, *I never knew him,* meant I didn't know a part of myself. Who knew all of that unresolved baggage sticks around until we decide to unpack it? If we don't unpack it, we'll eat it.

Inner Glutton Revealed

We went deeper.

"What other memories do you sense?" she asked after my stream of tears slowed.

"I'm six years old eating sauerkraut at my grandmother's house. I stuffed myself with it." An agonizing, heart-wrenching sob emerged, and choppy words persisted with an aha! moment, "Oh my goodness, my parents just got divorced. I had no one to talk to even though my family was right there!"

Kali handed me tissue after tissue for several minutes. She helped me to understand again my younger self believed she was defective. The divorce benefited my mom and dad but left me with a fear I'd be abandoned and rejected in intimate relationships.

I'd sauerkraut'ed my emotions that day to the point of vomiting. Until that moment, I was unaware of where my deep dependency on food began.

I worked with Kali and the Holy Spirit over time to reshape my thoughts and beliefs to internalize the truth; I'm never alone. God's always with me.

Emotional wounds drive emotional eating.

Childhood drama and its unpredictability gets recreated with inner drama with weight and eating. My little girl self at various ages needed to experience and release these emotions so I could successfully move forward to weight and eating freedom.

Binges contain messages about our identity. My Inner Glutton was my hurt little girl self that I had to embrace to heal.

I still had a lot of work to do, but I left her office a new woman.

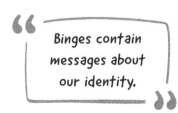

> Binges contain messages about our identity.

Healing Emotional Eating

Everyone emotionally eats. The question is to what degree? Is it a binge to the tune of 200 calories or 5,000? Does it happen multiple times per day or once in a blue moon?

Emotional eaters eat from an ***emotionally triggered*** place. That place is our emotional wounds. Emotions we'd rather not feel or aren't comfortable feeling, we manifest as a hearty lasagna, then eat our feelings masked by the lasagna.

My present situation, my husband's absence, triggered an *implosion*—an episode of Inner Glutton overeating. This particular episode I called, Death by Sticky Buns.

Our past impacts our present reactions and choices. To my surprise, the trigger of loneliness, which spurred an eating binge over my husband's absence, wasn't about my husband at all.

It was about unresolved pain from the same emotion of abandonment ungrieved by my father's absence. In other words, when I felt lonely or abandoned in the present, I ate from the past abandonment of my father.

My friends, this is the golden key to healing our emotional eating. We eat excess because Inner Glutton is an unhealed child within, trapped inside of an erroneous belief about who he or she is. Our child inside needs to be heard, loved, and affirmed by us, their caregiver. It takes processing difficult emotions to heal. And it's a tough to process without tools.

Out of the heart the mouth speaks (Luke 6:45b). And I say, out of the heart the mouth eats. Because in my episode, Death by Sticky Buns, I ate from the soul wound of abandonment. Once healed, I

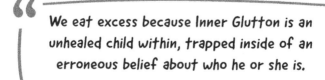

> We eat excess because Inner Glutton is an unhealed child within, trapped inside of an erroneous belief about who he or she is.

could no longer eat from or out of that emotional wound, because the abandonment of not knowing my dad was no longer *there* to eat from.

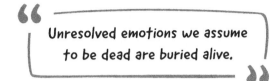

> Unresolved emotions we assume to be dead are buried alive.

Unresolved emotions we assume to be dead are buried alive.

For the first time in my life, I allowed myself to fully cry out my grief over my dad's death without holding back. And boy did I cry. I cried for hours, everywhere I went, for days!

After my consuming wonder of why on earth I hadn't made my emotional 911 call years sooner, a remarkable strategy birthed. *The Emotional Fitness Workout*™, a five step inner workout.

EMOTIONAL EATING STRONGHOLD QUIZ

Put a check next to the answer that describes your emotional strength and add the total points below. The higher the score, the more emotional wounds are present.

1. How often do you use food to alleviate negative emotions and stress?

☐ (5) ALWAYS ☐ (4) OFTEN ☐ (3) SOMETIMES ☐ (2) RARELY ☐ (1) NEVER

2. How often can you recognize emotions that sparked the reason(s) you used food?

☐ (1) ALWAYS ☐ (2) OFTEN ☐ (3) SOMETIMES ☐ (4) RARELY ☐ (5) NEVER

3. How often do you identify what you're feeling when you're feeling it?

☐ (1) ALWAYS ☐ (2) OFTEN ☐ (3) SOMETIMES ☐ (4) RARELY ☐ (5) NEVER

4. How often do you differentiate physical hunger from emotional hunger?

☐ (1) ALWAYS ☐ (2) OFTEN ☐ (3) SOMETIMES ☐ (4) RARELY ☐ (5) NEVER

5. How often do you divert your actions from harming yourself with food?

☐ (1) ALWAYS ☐ (2) OFTEN ☐ (3) SOMETIMES ☐ (4) RARELY ☐ (5) NEVER

6. How often do you take time to feel your feelings?

☐ (1) ALWAYS ☐ (2) OFTEN ☐ (3) SOMETIMES ☐ (4) RARELY ☐ (5) NEVER

7. How often do you judge or criticize the way you feel?

☐ (5) ALWAYS ☐ (4) OFTEN ☐ (3) SOMETIMES ☐ (2) RARELY ☐ (1) NEVER

8. How often do you blame your poor eating choices on how someone made you feel?

☐ (5) ALWAYS ☐ (4) OFTEN ☐ (3) SOMETIMES ☐ (2) RARELY ☐ (1) NEVER

9. How often do you make yourself feel better with things besides food?

☐ (1) ALWAYS ☐ (2) OFTEN ☐ (3) SOMETIMES ☐ (4) RARELY ☐ (5) NEVER

10. How often do you use a process or strategy to clear your negative emotions?

☐ (1) ALWAYS ☐ (2) OFTEN ☐ (3) SOMETIMES ☐ (4) RARELY ☐ (5) NEVER

Total Score:

Score Sheet
30–50 | You're in the right place!
20–30 | You've done some hard work and it shows!
10–20 | Handle this weight and eating thing and you're golden!

_____

What Are Emotions?

Miriam Webster describes emotion as a conscious mental reaction (such as anger or fear) subjectively experienced as strong feeling usually directed toward a specific object and typically accompanied by bodily physiological and behavioral changes.[1]

Emotions have the root word motion, which means action, and are intertwined with our thoughts, actions, and beliefs per Chapter 17. And while emotional states tend to be transient, what we do as a result of emotional eating sabotages our health. To graduate from emotional eating, we need to become emotionally savvy.

Your Choice to Become Emotionally Fit

Emotional healing is like a hotel in your soul. The more painful the past, the larger the number of rooms. These rooms carry labels, such as "rejected at sixteen at the school dance" or "criticized in front of friends by Mom" or "men." These times in your past shaped your mindsets and thoughts today.

You make the choice to open the door to each room and allow the Holy Spirit to come in and clean it out. After it's clean, the Holy Spirit fills it up with God's love and truth, then moves into another room as you unlock permission.

Before a miracle like what took place in Kali's office, my soul had to go through prep work. Along my journey, I found the book *Feelings Buried Alive Never Die* by Karol Truman.

It helped me realize that I gave my power to emotions, money, food, my mother, my circumstances—basically anything as an excuse to eat whatever I wanted despite the negative effects on my body.

We're victimized and tormented by emotional wounds until we deal with them.

Healing is a part of our spiritual path. Healing is the tough, real work of the mature. The more fruit

> *Healing is the tough, real work of the mature.*

233

of the Spirit evidenced in our lives, the more we know we've been healed (Galatians 5:22).

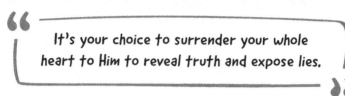

> It's your choice to surrender your whole heart to Him to reveal truth and expose lies.

It's up to you to invite the Holy Spirit into your healing. It's your choice to surrender your whole heart to Him to reveal truth and expose lies. This process is lifelong, there's no end date, but it gets easier.

We'll learn how to do the Emotional Fitness Workout™, then enact an Emotional Strength Training Plan to grow bigger than running to food like it's our grandmama with our emotional problems.

Will you make the choice to become emotionally fit?

What Is Emotional Fitness?

The five step Emotional Fitness Workout™ is a tool to help you process painful emotions that affect your emotional eating choices. Emotional fitness is your skill of what you feel, connected to why you feel that way. To strengthen our emotional body, reduces our need to protect and defend with chubby suits or Inner Glutton sabotage.

Emotional fitness strengthens the emotional body to handle offenses, upsets, disappointments, and overall feelings effectively when they occur so we're not eating over them. Wouldn't you love to get over an offense sooner? How about a disappointment in less than five minutes?

The power of emotional fitness is you get to take your power out of the hands of others, circumstances, and food. Emotional fitness for weight and eating strengthens your emotional body as a foundation for better physical and spiritual health.

When to Start an Emotional Fitness Workout™

Just as an alarm goes off to start your day, a trigger is the alarm to start an Emotional Fitness Workout.™

We Know We're Triggered When

- We have an overwhelming urge to find food. We seek out fast food, raid the kitchen cabinets, run to the convenience store for junk food, or tap into a secret stash of candy.
- We feel strong emotions such as loneliness, defeat, anger, grief, guilt, and/or embarrassment. We may also feel fat or ugly.
- We feel fearful, unsafe, threatened, or uncomfortable (chubbological triggers).
- We shut down all emotions, numb them, and isolate with excess screen time (the Internet, movies, television, or social media) and mindless eating.
- We're about to overeat, want to overeat, or have just overeaten.
- We're sabotaging progress, regaining weight, and/or choosing poorly.

Have any of these signs affected you in the past week? Moving forward, look for signs that you've been triggered and start the Emotional Fitness Workout.™

THE EMOTIONAL FITNESS WORKOUT™	
Step #1: Stop	How can I disengage in self-harming pursuits?
Step #2: Pinpoint	What triggered me and what emotions am I feeling exactly?
Step #3: Evaluate	Why am I feeling this way?
Step #4: Experience	How can I best process my feelings right now?
Step #5: Release	What or who do I need to let go of?

Step 1 – Stop

How can I disengage in self-harming pursuits?

"Stop," the officer said, "Put the knife and fork down." Couldn't you use the food police from time to time to help you put excess food down? The first step in the Emotional Fitness Workout™ is to stop. To stop is to consciously disengage your Inner Glutton when he or she's tempted to excessively eat. This step strengthens your emotional impulse control muscle.

- Ben cruised angrily down the road after work. He pulled up to Wendy's drive through, as he savored the number 4 combo. By the time his turn came at the window, he drove away.

- Amanda knew if she bought the chocolate cake, she'd eat it all. She walked past the bakery section and continued grocery shopping.

- Tina crunched the corner of a tortilla chip, then threw it and the rest of the bag out. She caught herself before the whole bag ended up featured on her belly.

- Sarah stared at the banana bread while home alone. She went outside to get fresh air to ward off the desire to devour it.

In the above examples, each person practiced step one. Like a Corvette can go from zero to sixty miles per hour in about three seconds, so too can our negative emotions drive us to food.

Before we look up, our Inner Glutton has already acted, and we're throwing out candy cartons. "She's quick," a Whole & Free Health course participant admitted, "Sometimes Inner Glutton's so fast I didn't even see what happened."

We turn to food as fast as we flip on a light switch. *Switch* and you've derailed your efforts. To stop, is to slow down the process from trigger point to an emotional eating episode.

As we increase our emotional pain tolerance, we gain impulse control. When we stop the behavior, we find reasons behind what's driving it. Next time think through what's going on behind the compulsion. This skill and first step is the hardest skill to learn, be gracious with yourself.

Ben didn't want to stop, no one really does, but he realized if he kept surrendering to his cravings telling him to get a burger, he'd get the same high blood pressure, frustration with his burger belly, and intimacy issues with his wife. All of which, came from his stops for fast food.

He needed to change. If it wasn't now, it would be later. Per his doctor, one more bite could propel him into a heart attack. Ben's eaten hundreds of fatty burgers in his forty years. When was enough, enough?

Aren't you inspired every time you choose life?

Emotional Pain Tolerance

> As we increase our emotional pain tolerance, we gain impulse control.

As Peter Scazzero says for the subtitle of his book *Emotionally Healthy Spirituality*, "It's impossible to be spiritually mature while remaining emotionally immature."[2]

We're to increase our emotional pain tolerance, and we can only do this with practice. A low emotional pain tolerance is guaranteed to throw us into the arms of a soft pretzel whenever we don't get what we want.

A low emotional pain tolerance thrives on self-destruction. When you stop the damage, your self-confidence increases. Would Ben have felt better or worse about himself if he had eaten fatty fast food? Each time we stop, we strengthen the "yes, I can do this" belief muscle.

Every time you succeed at step one, you rebuild from the demoralization you've taught yourself over the years by breaking your own agreements. Instead of saying yes to self-harm, self-destruction, and shame, you can say "yes!" to your true identity.

To strengthen the most difficult emotional muscle of all, impulse control, allows us to learn delayed gratification—also known as the spiritual practice of patience. Our flesh loves to get what it wants when it wants, but this very nature is anti-progress.

As long time emotional eaters, we'll always make excuses and rationalize eating more. Always! Food is how we cope. Food is our favorite reward. It's our default modus of operandi.

How to Stop

To stop, do the following:

- **Pray.** Try simple prayers like, "Spirit, I need your help right now to stop my compulsion to go to food. Please help me to stop and do the right thing in this moment."
- **Reflect on three reasons you want to stop from your Action Plan.** Ben reflected on his biggest reasons:
  1. I want to love God with all of my heart, soul, and strength, not food.
  2. I want to see my children grow up.
  3. I want to pay for one airline seat, not two.

- **Cheerlead yourself to stop.** Ben said to himself, *I can do this. My boss isn't worth more negative health reports. I can drive home and eat leftovers. I can change. The same power that raised Jesus from the dead lives in me.*
- **Think about three negative consequences of chubby choices.** Give thought to the repercussions of poor decisions. The consequences of our choices must become harder to swallow. These are the opposite of what you want.

Ben's negative consequences were clear:

1. I'll dishonor my temple.
2. I won't reverse heart disease.
3. I could risk not seeing my daughter grow into a woman and walking her down the aisle when she gets married.

- **Speak to the food itself.** Ben spoke to the food temptation directly, with attitude. He said, "Number 4 burger you're not my god. I let you go." It does help to say "stop!" out loud, too.

  You have the power of the Holy Spirit inside of you to stop the impulsivity to go to food when emotional. So, when fast food screams your name, use it.

What If You Can't Stop?

You can stop before, during, or after going to food. Once you stop, go onto step two. But sometimes, we can't stop. This happens when we're overcome by something physiological, such as food addiction or when the emotion is deeply rooted. Be patient with yourself and move on to step two to support uncovering the source of the binge.

REFLECT & SHARE

1. What foods do you go to when you have a negative emotional reaction?

   _____

2. What have you done in the past to stop a chubby choice?

   _____

3. From the ideas above, what's one thing you can do when triggered to emotionally eat?

   _____

Step 2 – Pinpoint
What triggered me and what emotions am I feeling exactly?

Whether you succeed at step one or not, implement step two. Step two, pinpoint, is recognizing your trigger(s) and emotions to strengthen your emotional literacy muscle to find the emotions you've been eating from.

Think about your last emotional eating episode. What made you want to eat in the first place? Whatever the answer—a fight with your adult child, a surprising performance review, or a break up—we call this a trigger.

Figure out what happened. Then ask yourself, what am I feeling?

- Ben had a tough past two years of reporting to Aaron. Aaron, a demanding and egotistical type, couldn't help but blast Ben in front of the team. Ben recognized his trigger was Aaron's words in front of other colleagues.

    Aaron said, "Ben, you're late and inconsistent. This report is not up to standards for our client. You need to redo this before next Tuesday."

    Ben pulled away from the drive through window as he recognized his anger toward Aaron. Ben pinpointed his feelings. Underneath Aaron's harsh words, Ben felt undermined and humiliated.

- For some time, Amanda craved chocolate cake after romantic dinners with her husband of forty years. The chocolate cake obsession after dinner was replacing Amanda's deep grief from unresolved pain of how terribly her husband treated her in the first three decades of their marriage. To stop the desire for chocolate cake's comfort meant processing the emotions of hurt, betrayal, and grief from her husband's numerous affairs, as well as the lost years of happiness she'd never get back.

- Marie discovered her excessive ice cream binges at night were triggered by financial stress. She was underpaid and wasn't eligible for promotion. Her anxiety caused her to eat over fear of her financial future.

We need to know what spurred the food reaction, then embrace our emotions without judgment.

When you're looking for a store in the mall you find on the map the red dot that says, "You are here". To pinpoint your emotions is to figure out where you are emotionally. Emotional literacy is an important step toward emotional fitness. We need to be able to put a name to the way we're feeling.

Like my father's story, which represented only a sliver of the wounds I emotionally ate from, we're emotionally stunted until we deal with it. These wounds don't just go away. We must decide *to feel them and heal them*. And we can't do that until we know how to identify them.

> **Emotional literacy is an important step toward emotional fitness.**

How to Pinpoint

To pinpoint, do the following:

- **Find your trigger.** Ideally, we have a clear scenario that compels us to eat. Figure out what that scenario is. If you tend to have a fast paced life or feel it's difficult to process emotions, consider everything happening in your life, then consider where there might be emotional charge to explore.

- **Study emotional vocabulary.** Most people identify about ten emotions they feel on a consistent basis, but there are 34,000 emotions.[3] Growing your emotional literacy also grows your emotional strength. Check out names of various emotions online.

- **Name your feelings.** You're not limited to one feeling. You can have five feelings happen at once. You can have a new feeling you haven't experienced before. Learn what your emotions are trying to tell you.

The most common places we're eating from are:

- **Anger**. Anger can also feel like injustice, resentment, disrespect, betrayal, or contempt.
- **Grief**. Grief can also feel like sadness, dejection, defeat, despair, loneliness, or abandonment.
- **Guilt**. Guilt can also feel like regret, sadness, anger, or fear.
- **Shame**. Shame can also feel like embarrassment, rejection, guilt, self-doubt, or insecurity.
- **Fear**. Fear can also feel like worry, anxiety, uncertainty, incompetency, or inadequacy.
- **Boredom**. Boredom can also feel like emptiness, meaninglessness, purposelessness, or restlessness.
- **Ambivalence**. Ambivalence can also feel like anxiety, insecurity, stagnation, pressure, or avoidance.
- **Overwhelm**. Overwhelm can also feel like insufficiency, fear, loss of control, or numbness.

According to Myers' Briggs Type Indicator, a personality assessment with years of indepth research on how people process emotions, people are classified to varying degrees as thinkers or feelers.[4] For thinker types that make decisions more objectively than subjectively, emotions can be difficult.

So, thinkers may take a day or two to realize what emotions they're feeling. I'm this type of person, which is why I had to do extra work to heal my emotional body. Stay hopeful. As you rehearse your last food binge episode, you'll find insights and connect the dots.

REFLECT & SHARE

1. What triggered you in your last binge?

_____

_____

2. How exactly did you feel about the situation?

_____

_____

Step 3 – Evaluate

Why am I feeling this way?

To evaluate, is to find causal reasons to your emotional button and connect the past to the present. After you identify what you're feeling and what happened that may have caused the feelings, ask yourself, "Why am I feeling this way?" or "When have I felt this way before?"

Wendy Backland, author of *Victorious Emotions*, says, "Emotions do not validate truth; they validate what we believe." She goes on to say, "We need to understand there's a difference between what we want to believe and what we subconsciously believe."[5]

To evaluate our emotions we're getting to what we believe consciously and subconsciously.

- As Ben evaluated his trigger, a memory came to mind of his teenage self.

  In the memory, Ben, his dad, and his brother Mark were in the garage. As Mark and Ben worked on a toy plane, Ben shared his idea to paint the plane burgundy.

Ben tested the burgundy paint on the wing. Ben's dad's alcoholic anger spiraled out of control, and in a split second, the atmosphere went from peaceful to hostile.

"Ben, why'd you do that?! So stupid!" Ben's dad slapped the plane wing off and raged out of the garage.

Ben and Mark followed, crushed.

Ben remembered the shattering he felt in his soul that day. He was older than Mark, and Mark looked up to Ben. Nonetheless, Ben's dad had the habit of having these outbursts in front of Mark. Aaron's rude outburst about Ben's performance hit a button in Ben's emotional body of feeling undermined.

- Tina argued with her husband. Afterwards, she typically ate a bag of tortilla chips to stuff the anger down. She discovered her trigger in a session. When Tina took extra care to dress up for her husband, he didn't offer her any positive affirmation of her beauty, even though she was stunning.

  His lack of validation stirred up arguments about trivial things. She longed for his words of affirmation like, "You're beautiful" or "You look great tonight, honey." But instead, her seething anger drew her to chips and guac while her husband got the silent treatment.

  Tina wondered, "Why wouldn't he give me a kind word when he knows that's my love language?!"

  After evaluating, Tina recalled memories of her mother never being validated by her father. It seemed the family had some sort of curse of beauty without validation.

  She also remembered a time when she dressed up in a beautiful ballerina outfit at age five. Her dad was interested in television more than in her. She twirled to get his attention, but he stubbornly watched television and ignored her beauty and twirls.

  Tina's hurt created emotional wounds of being unvalidated, not pretty enough, and unworthy of attention. She needed to process her feelings to forgive her husband and dad for not validating her beauty.

- Sarah processed through her emotions and found a memory where she came home from school and ate candy and junk food to the point of sickness in her room while watching television. She ate the loneliness away. She ate away the belief that she wasn't wanted.

After you take time to figure out what emotions you're feeling, evaluate all the reasons you're experiencing them. This is figured out best by questioning yourself in what I call *episode interrogation*. Perform one until you find a connection from the past to the present.

Be prayerful in the evaluating process. The Spirit knows all.

How to Evaluate

To evaluate, do the following:

- **Perform an episode interrogation.** Ask yourself the following questions to reveal the root of the emotion or the memories about how you're feeling.

  1. Why do I feel this way?
  2. When have I felt this way before?
  3. When is my earliest memory of feeling this way?
  4. What am I saying to myself?
  5. What am I afraid of? What's the worst that can happen?
  6. What am I believing right now that's making me feel or behave this way?
  7. Why am I so offended?

- **Find the root memory.** Ask "locate the source" of the emotions you're feeling. Memories such as pictures, thoughts, words, or past situations may seem disconnected at first, but are a part of the answer in locating the source.

- **Talk it out with a good friend, family member, or your accountability partner.** The act of sharing our emotional self can help to evaluate and experience our feelings.

WHOLE & FREE HEALTH

REFLECT & SHARE

1. What memories from your past are connected with your present eating episode?

_____

_____

2. Perform an episode interrogation from your last emotional eating event. What did you discover?

_____

_____

Step 4 – Experience

How can I best process my feelings right now?

Up until now, you've judged, criticized, and condemned your emotions. You've made excuses to eat over them. And you may even wallow in them during lonely weekends as you couple up with cookies, or at least I did.

Feeling has been difficult.

You've numbed yourself with food and other things that may have allowed you to escape emotions. But the true test of our healing is our willingness and ability to feel our feelings instead of eating them. Step 4 is all about feeling your feelings. And we won't be able to skirt this with an emoji.

- Ben processed his anger toward Aaron while driving home. He spoke out what he would've said if he could've said it without getting fired.

"Aaron, you're a bad boss! I hate having you as a boss. How dare you speak to me like that in front of my colleagues?! I'm sick and tired of you undermining my authority and talent! You're a jerk! The Green report was good enough! You just want to nitpick and look for things to harass me about!"

Ben went on for half of his thirty five minute commute home. So what if the other drivers on the road thought he was a nut case. Ben felt good about getting the anger out of him.

- Tina wrote her husband a letter to express her frustration about him not validating her beauty. Through writing out how angry and hurt she felt, she released words stuffed down with tortilla chips. She then prayed for herself and her mother to release the anger about not feeling validated. Tina didn't give her husband the letter.

- Marie sat with the deep fear of not being able to cover her bills. She continued to process her emotions and discovered a link to her childhood poverty. It was difficult as a child to get what she wanted. She made the connection from her present financial anxiety to her past financial poverty.

> But the true test of our healing is our willingness and ability to feel our feelings instead of eating them.

Underneath the mountain of difficult emotions like anger, fear, or grief is a great reservoir of love and joy. But to attain emotional treasures you've got to process your feelings. Feeling your feelings on the front end will reduce your body's backend.

Because we're body, soul, and spirit, we know there are emotional causes that need to be addressed, since what's toxic physically or emotionally will manifest.

As Peter Scazzero says, "To minimize or distort what we feel is a distortion of what it means to be image bearers of God." And, "to the degree that we're unable to express our emotions, we remain impaired in our ability to love God, others, and ourselves well."[5] I couldn't agree more.

How To Experience

To experience, do the following:

- **Sit still.** Sit with your feelings. You may find a need to pray, cry, or scream. All is acceptable. Turn off the distractions, quiet all noise, and be with your own soul. Emotions surface as you get quiet. If you have family in the house, ask for alone time, sit in your car, or reserve a room at the library.

  The seas of feeling can feel choppy at first, but I promise an emotional shark won't devour you. You'll get good at exercising your emotional body. What we do is avoid feeling by eating because we think it's so hard to feel, but then we deal with the hardship of our poor choices. So, go ahead, bust out the tissues and skip the shenanigans.

- **Heal the memory.** When a memory comes up for you, speak the truth to it.

  - Speak to the younger version of yourself in the memory and say what you needed to hear at the time. Be kind and gentle. Tina spoke the validation she needed to her five-year-old self, "You're so pretty! Look at you! You're beautiful!"

  - Speak the truth to others involved. Say what you've wanted to say, even if it's ugly. This can be done on paper. Tina confronted her dad, "I'm much more interesting than the television. You should've given me a word of affirmation. I needed it as your little girl. Because I didn't get your affirmation, I looked for it wrongly from men!"

  - Allow a greater positive memory to be imagined. Tina imagined what her dad should've done and said to her when she came into the living room dressed up as a ballerina. She allowed herself to feel the joy and excitement of his imagined validation and affirmation.

- **Write a letter directly to the situation.** When angry, you can write directly to who or what you're angry at. It can be sugar addiction, your spouse, yourself, your job, or the scale. You can write a letter to a rock! Deal with it directly on paper. This helps you to clarify your feelings to understand yourself in the matter. When angry or upset, write a letter directly to the person or circumstance that's making you upset. Tell them directly your raw feelings and thoughts. Do not give the person the letter.

- **Speak it out loud.** If you don't enjoy writing, speaking it out loud has the same results. Like Ben in his car, speak to the issue directly. It's healthy to learn how to express yourself in less awkward, rude, and passive aggressive ways. When you speak it out, you'll get words to interact healthier in person.

- **Journal.** Journaling is the best way I find to process emotions. Journaling on a consistent basis has been instrumental in my process because journals are a place to share freely. If you're concerned about someone finding your journals, find a secret place to store them.

- **Hit something.** An anger workout was popular in the 70s and involves getting your anger out honestly by using a plastic bat against the sofa and screaming out what you're upset about as though you're talking directly to the person or problem.

  You can yell into a paper bag or stomp and scream. While this may be nutty to onlookers, you'll be the doing a happy dance that those ugly emotions are out of your heart.

It's Your Human Right to Feel

The human heart is the seat of emotions, and it's the truest part of you. In emotional fitness, we look at how we can speak the truth of our heart for healing.

The greatest stories ever written are filled with emotion.
Feeling is your human right.

To devalue or repress them, as Peter Scazzero says, is also to deny being "human and made in the image of God."[7] Embrace your humanness for a whole and free life in Christ.

> **Feeling is your human right.**

REFLECT & SHARE

1. How do you procrastinate feeling?

_____

_____

_____

2. What feelings are you uncomfortable with experiencing?

_____

_____

_____

3. Pick a technique for feeling your feelings and try it on your last emotional eating episode.

_____

_____

_____

Step 5 – Release

What or who do I need to let go of?

By definition, to release is to allow (a person or animal) to leave a jail, cage, prison, etc.; to set (someone or something) free; to stop holding (someone or something).[8]

- To release Aaron would free Ben from the resentment that drove him to Wendy's. Ben followed the steps and released the three parties that were held in contempt in Ben's heart: Aaron, his dad, and himself.

  He parked the car in the driveway of his suburban home.

  Okay, I can do this, he thought to himself. "Aaron, I release you from my judgments against you—for being rude, inconsiderate, undermining me, and being disrespectful to me in front of my colleagues. Because of your words, I felt hurt, rejected, embarrassed, ashamed, and undermined. God is the Judge, and I forgive you fully and completely. I will honor you and respect you in spite of how you have treated me. Aaron, I let you go. God bless you and forgive me for my resentment and judgments."

  He was on a roll, "Dad, I release you from my judgments against you—for being a horrible dad, for being abusive, harsh, and mocking me in front of Mark. You made me feel hurt, angry, disrespected, embarrassed, and dishonored. I'll honor you and respect you in spite of how you've treated me. God bless you and forgive me for my resentment and judgments."

  Ben took a deep breath and looked into the drop-down mirror.

  "Ben, I release you from my judgments against you—for your lack of thoroughness in the Green report, for not standing up for yourself, for being a coward, for going to food to help you, and for not preventing that situation with a third review. You should know by now what Aaron wants. You made yourself feel undermined, stupid, disrespected, angry, resentful, upset, and targeted. I forgive you."

  Ben felt an inner release as his ten-year-old son ran out from their house to see what his old man was talking to himself about. Ben, relieved and proud, grabbed his computer bag, locked up the car, and hugged his boy. "I love you, son."

- Tina made the executive life decision that she would validate herself. After writing letters to her husband and father, she wrote one to herself to let go of her need for affirmation from anyone else. She was free. Shortly thereafter, her husband and others started complimenting her on a frequent basis. The underlying resentment was resolved. She released her husband, and the crazy cravings for chips and guac were a distant memory.

- Marie let go of her financial worry by turning it into positive actions. Instead of eating ice cream, she put her energy into changing her financial story. She texted friends for job openings, looked into getting a bachelor's degree, and updated her resume over the next several nights. Action in the right direction took the cravings away.

> Spirit is the leader when it comes to processing and releasing emotions.

Forgiveness Restores

We want to be in a constant state of forgiveness. We're also to forgive the man in the mirror, as we hold ourselves in much condemnation and contempt over our chubby choices.

Practice the art of forgiveness and receive the scientific benefits as well. A study of married couples showed that when the victim in the situation forgave the other person *both* experienced lower blood pressure.[9] And *not* forgiving someone is associated with more anger, anxiety, and sadness.[10]

Spiritually, to release is also beneficial.

You may wonder, what if a heinous act was committed, such as rape or incest? How do you forgive in situations like that? Process your emotions and ultimately release until you feel peace.

Forgiveness doesn't mean you agree with the act that was done.

But to stay victimized, the perpetrator still has power over your life, because holding onto unforgiveness is like eating a cream-filled donut on a regular basis and expecting the other person to buy the bigger underwear.

Make the tough decision to forgive in all circumstances, in advance. The *fore* in forgive, means beforehand. When we release our needs or the people involved, we take back our health.

> Holding onto unforgiveness is like eating a cream-filled donut on a regular basis and expecting the other person to buy the bigger underwear.

How to Release

To release do the following:

- **Get clear.** First clarify what you need to let go. Ask:
  - Who or what do I need to let go of?
  - Where do I feel "right" or judgmental?
  - What do I think about myself, my circumstance, or the person (people) involved?
  - What emotion do I need to let go of?

- **Speak it out.** Like Ben's example, confess aloud or write I forgive you (person or thing) for (what you feel they did, how they are, and how you judge them) and making me feel (your feelings about it). Be as descriptive as possible.

- **Write a thank you letter to the situation or person upsetting you.** Thank them for all the positive things they've done for you. This fosters forgiveness and perspective.

- **Write the rest of the story.** Create a narrative of yourself in the midst of the circumstance or situation that you're dealing with. Write it as though a story and finish the story with a better ending.

- **Remember to forgive yourself.** Heal your emotions and the pain caused by your own acts of stupidity, overeating, indulgence, or whatever else. We all make significant mistakes, it's an undeniable fact of the human experience, forgive it, and move on with your life.
- **Look in the mirror.** Do the work above in the mirror. It adds a layer of healing you can only get looking into your own eyes. Try it.
- **Take action.** One thing we may need to release is our inaction or wallowing in the emotions. Because emotions stir action, what actions do you need to take next? What actions can support a better decision?

  Instead of eating over what's eating you, take action in a positive direction. Make a list of actions that would relieve you from negative emotions. You may need to have a conversation with someone to resolve things fully or figure out how to do something you've never done. But get to work. And, remember prayer is an action, too.

REFLECT & SHARE

1. What triggers/buttons cause you to overeat?

   _____

   _____

2. How often does this happen?

   _____

   _____

3. What can you do to prevent the button/trigger?

   _____

   _____

Your Emotional Strength Training Plan
What triggers can I heal before they happen?

An **Emotional Strength Training Plan** is the practice of emotionally clearing and completing Emotional Fitness Workouts™ when triggered. Your emotional chub gets ripped by being intentional about strengthening your emotional body.

To enact an Emotional Strength Training Plan, do the following consistently:

1. **Complete an Emotional Fitness Workout™ as soon as you feel triggered.** Practice the five steps to fully process your emotions and heal the button being triggered. You'll get really good at it, and people around you will notice your change on the inside and the outside.

2. **Emotionally Clear.** Often once a day or every few days, complete an emotionally clearing exercise. Grab a pen or ponder the responses. You can even say, "In regard to life …" or "In regard to my marriage …" or "In regard to my weight …" to dig up and clear more negative feelings.

   • I feel mad because …

   • I feel sad because …

   • I feel glad because …

   • I feel bad because …

3. **Get good at identifying your buttons.** Put language to the trigger that causes an emotional over-reaction or impulse by writing them down. List the things that currently upset you or give you the urge to eat.

4. **Hire a therapist to work through your emotions.** One study found that 190 overweight or obese persons lost on average 13 percent of body weight over the course of a year by using acceptance-based therapy methods.[11] Dialectical Behavioral Therapy (DBT) helped

40 percent of participants release weight in a twenty week study receiving treatment and materials, versus only 3.3 percent of the wait list who didn't receive support.[12]

Other studies show that Cognitive Behavioral Therapy (CBT) supported a 5 to 8 percent reduction in body weight over the course of the year.[13] Either way, many studies show that psychotherapy positively affects your personal health and wellbeing. Therapists also help you process difficult feelings.[14]

5. **Keep learning about emotions.** Books mentioned: *Feelings Buried Alive Never Die* by Karol Truman, *Victorious Emotions* by Wendy Buckland, or *Emotionally Healthy Spirituality* by Peter Scazzero help our knowledge and wisdom in healing the emotional body. Also look out for my upcoming book *Emotional Fitness for Spiritual Strength.*

6. **Boost your mood to gain a better perspective.** To boost your mood after processing through negative emotions try the following strategies to switch to a more positive emotional channel.

- **Listen to music.** Music can increase feel good neurotransmitters to elevate your emotional state in minutes. Put on your favorite music and dance like David danced for an even greater effect.

- **Take a hot bath.** It helps muscles and the soul relax.

- **Exercise.** We covered this in Habit 5. Nothing beats a natural anti-depressant like exercise. Go for a walk.

- **Attend church or an inspirational program.** You don't have to leave home to find some motivation and inspiration on YouTube. Tune in to your favorite televangelists online.

- **Pray for those you love.** Praying for others helps us to move through our own upsets, and gets us into a more benevolent frame of mind.

Encouragement

When we choose to do this soul work, inner breakthroughs become a part of the adventure of living life with God.

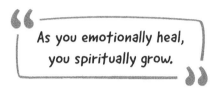

As you emotionally heal, you spiritually grow.

Emotional eating episodes become less frequent and calorically destructive. As you emotionally heal, you spiritually grow. And, as you emotionally heal, you physically improve your health.

But just like you can't run a mile this week and expect to be fit for a marathon next week, the same is true here. Emotional strength isn't built in a day. It's built from years of doing Emotional Fitness Workouts™ trigger after trigger, button after button, until very few, if any, buttons can be pressed.

An Emotional S.P.E.E.R.

An acronym for the steps is: S.P.E.E.R. When triggered, take a spear (SPEER) to kill emotional eating at the root.

S: Stop
P: Pinpoint
E: Evaluate
E: Experience
R: Release

Alrighty, take a few minutes to memorize it.

This workout does for the emotional body what exercise does for the physical body and what the prayer does for the spiritual body. When you're triggered, don't let it fester. As often as you can, get to the bottom of your emotional eating pit.

Take your healing process one day, one hour, and one moment at a time. Implement the Emotional Fitness Workout™ frequently. I remember as I worshipped God one morning, I thought, *How will I ever get through this? Will I ever overcome?* Never forget, we're overcomers. And we'll be whole and free, inch by inch, insight by insight, step by step, skill by skill.

REFLECT & SHARE

1. What step in the Emotional Fitness Workout™ is most difficult for you? Why?

_____

_____

_____

_____

_____

_____

2. What emotions do you need to process?

_____

_____

_____

_____

_____

_____

CHAPTER 19

LOOKSOLOGY
JUMP OFF THE BODY SHAME TRAIN

*"God gave me my body. I just added to it,
enhanced it if you will."* —Chubby Church member

I carried a giant stack of textbooks like a football into my seventh grade English class. My crush, Richard, walked into the class with me when we heard, "You jolly green giant," shouted from the hallway. "Is that Nikki B.?" I asked as I felt the heat in my face.

Earlier that day, I heard that Nikki was the one who spread horrible rumors about me, causing conflict with my friends. She said I had said derogatory things, which I didn't say. I know because I'm not one to gossip or talk about people like that. I just never liked it. So, all that had been said was indeed a lie. I was ready for her. I just wasn't ready for her attack on my height.

I was about 5'9" by the time I was in seventh grade, and although I didn't wear green, the Jolly Green Giant — canned vegetable mascot — triggered my body shame.

Richard came to my defense. "She's just jealous," he said.

I was tickled by his quick defense, but jealous or not, my rage swung me full force into the hallway where I wacked her upside the forehead and grabbed the top of her big hair into a ponytail. Then with Hulk Hogan strength I picked her up by her hair and dangled her there against the wall for a few seconds.

"I'm sorry. I'm sorry!" she said between sobs. I dropped her onto the floor and then gave her a good kick or five before a teacher stopped the madness and broke up the crowd.

All of this happened one handed because the stack of books had my right hand securing it. We were sent to detention where we made up and were cordial for the rest of our school years.

I didn't get into fights often. I was a sweet girl and minded my own business. But she underestimated a fatherless daughter with a chaotic, deprived homelife. At the time I felt justified because I was triggered by her attack on my height in front of my crush, nonetheless.

In hindsight body shame, not Nikki, deserved a good whack upside the head.

Let me tell you another story about body shame that's not riddled in teenage girl drama and is much more spiritually mature.

My aunt and I snapped photos at the *Route 1* scenic area in Key West, Florida, and came across a man and his wife in their late forties. I overheard his wife's complaints about her looks as she prepared to take photos of him alone.

"Hey, I'm happy to take your photo together," I said as I sensed something more.

"I don't take photos," she said. I could see the shame in her eyes.

"She doesn't take photos," her husband reiterated. I could see the sadness in his.

"I'm so ashamed of my weight. I can't stand taking photos," she confessed.

"How long has she been like this about photos," I asked her husband.

"Since I've known her, maybe thirteen years," he said, "It's been a real struggle. I have hundreds of photos by myself or with the kids. See," he showed us his cell phone.

My aunt and I leaned in as he swiped through dozens of photos of only himself. His beautiful wife felt she wasn't picture worthy because she didn't weigh the same as she did in high school.

I felt the warmth of the Holy Spirit come upon me as I turned toward her and said, "Do you have any idea how beautiful you are? When you're ninety, you'll wish you had the youth you do now and a photo to prove it, right?" we chuckled. "More importantly, your children and great grandchildren will long for the photos of their beloved matriarch."

My soap box didn't end there. I am the author of *The Chubby Church* after all. I continued, "Weight will go when you stop obeying its shame. You've been shaming your body and hating how you look, but has it helped? Love God. Love yourself. Love your body. And the weight will follow."

With wet eyes she admitted, "I see my daughter struggle too, yet she's so beautiful."

Gently I responded, "Yes, beautiful like her mother. Where do you think she got this struggle from? Body shame has plagued your family long enough, hasn't it? Don't you want to make memories? And seriously, have you seen some of the folks on the beach?" I said with a funny face to make her smile. We chuckled as we glanced in the direction of glaring suspects who shamelessly let it all, and I mean all, hang out.

"I wish I were one of them," she giggled as she wiped her tears.

"You can be. You can be free. Jesus already did it," I said.

"I believe Him. He spoke to me about my body shame issues just this morning! I can't believe you're saying this to me," she admitted.

"Well, that explains why I'm able to speak freely to you," my hands gestured her over to the *Route 1* sign as I said, "I'm taking your photo."

I took a photo of her and her husband together for the first time in a long time. A memory they'd never forget.

"Thank you," they both said at the same time as all of our eye ducts swelled. He put his arm around his beautiful wife tightly and prepared for the photo that broke the bondage of body shame.

"Smile!" I said with a big grin. *Click. Click. Click.*

Is Your Body Relationship Adversarial?

Do you resonate with this woman? Do you beat up your body with harsh punches of criticism? Does how you feel about your body affect how you live your life?

I deeply empathize.

Before I could ever speak with that lady, I had to recognize and heal the distorted image of my own body. And despite weight reduction, my mind's body glasses needed new lenses.

We must win this battle because negative body evaluation, the technical term for not liking your body, is not only the common thread in all eating disorders but a strong causal factor to developing one.[1]

> "Any dysfunctional, adversarial relationship with food reflects a dysfunctional, adversarial relationship with our bodies."

Any dysfunctional, adversarial relationship with food reflects a dysfunctional, adversarial relationship with our bodies. How we feel about our bodies predicts and influences our weight and eating behaviors.[2]

Body shame is to hold our bodies and looks in contempt because we think we should look better or different. Our harsh judgments cause our self-esteem to crumble under the pressure placed on our looks, weight, and other physical attributes.

This battle is as fierce as food addiction and overeating.

In Part One: Understanding Body Shame of this chapter, we'll gain understanding about body shame, and in Part Two: Win the Body Shame Battle.

> "Body shame is to hold our bodies and looks in contempt because we think we should look better or different."

Let's take a quiz to see exactly where you stand in the battle of body shame.

BODY SHAME STRONGHOLD QUIZ

Put a check next to the answer that describes your body relationship and add the total points below. The higher the score the more body shame is present.

1. How often do you need validation around your looks or appearance?

☐ (5) ALWAYS ☐ (4) OFTEN ☐ (3) SOMETIMES ☐ (2) RARELY ☐ (1) NEVER

2. How often do you avoid looking in the mirror?

☐ (5) ALWAYS ☐ (4) OFTEN ☐ (3) SOMETIMES ☐ (2) RARELY ☐ (1) NEVER

3. How often do you grab, pick, pinch, tug, or pull at your body parts in disgust?

☐ (5) ALWAYS ☐ (4) OFTEN ☐ (3) SOMETIMES ☐ (2) RARELY ☐ (1) NEVER

4. How often do you excessively check your perceived flaws in mirrors?

☐ (5) ALWAYS ☐ (4) OFTEN ☐ (3) SOMETIMES ☐ (2) RARELY ☐ (1) NEVER

5. How often do you use makeup or clothing (all black, revealing, or over-sized) to hide your feelings of ugliness, inadequacy, discomfort, or shame around your face or body?

☐ (5) ALWAYS ☐ (4) OFTEN ☐ (3) SOMETIMES ☐ (2) RARELY ☐ (1) NEVER

6. How often do you get plastic surgery or treatments to improve your looks?

☐ (5) ALWAYS ☐ (4) OFTEN ☐ (3) SOMETIMES ☐ (2) RARELY ☐ (1) NEVER

7. How often do you avoid going out because of feeling fat/or overwhelmed by insecurities?

☐ (5) ALWAYS ☐ (4) OFTEN ☐ (3) SOMETIMES ☐ (2) RARELY ☐ (1) NEVER

8. How often do you scrutinize or comment on the weight, shape, or body parts of others?

☐ (5) ALWAYS ☐ (4) OFTEN ☐ (3) SOMETIMES ☐ (2) RARELY ☐ (1) NEVER

9. How often do you assume others talk about your perceived physical flaws?

☐ (5) ALWAYS ☐ (4) OFTEN ☐ (3) SOMETIMES ☐ (2) RARELY ☐ (1) NEVER

10. How often do you refuse to take photos or have them posted on social media?

☐ (5) ALWAYS ☐ (4) OFTEN ☐ (3) SOMETIMES ☐ (2) RARELY ☐ (1) NEVER

Total Score:

_____

Date:

_____

Score Sheet

30–50 | Your body deserves a raise in love tokens!

20–30 | You're learning how to accept your body, nice job!

10–20 | You're exiting the body shame train.

What Is Body Image?

A healthy body image reflects who we are because how we look is a profound identifier of who we are. The way we look is the truest form of ID. Nothing says you more than your face. Your face and body are both a picture of the soul and a mirror to it.

We get to see the invisible soul through the visible body.

> **We get to see the invisible soul through the visible body.**

A healthy body relationship allows us to feel good in the skin we're in and take care of it. Confident. Bold. Even if we're wearing our chubby suit, we're not bound or hidden in it because a healthy body relationship allows us to be more willing to go places, do things, reach our goals, and take risks.

Body image is multidimensional like weight. How we look holds societal importance and impacts our perceived self-worth. Multiple studies show that body image influences our self-esteem, sexual intimacy, work confidence, health, eating decisions, and mood.[3] Body image also affects how well or how poorly we treat the body as sacred. Hello, body imagine impacts every area of our lives.

Body image is made up of four areas:[4]

1. How we perceive our bodies visually

2. How we feel about our physical appearance

3. How we think and talk to ourselves about our bodies

4. Our sense of how other people view our bodies

Do you feel driven to be thin or muscular? Do you hate looking in the mirror? Most of us have what body image activist Dr. Renee Engeln, PhD, calls "beauty sickness," which she describes as the syndrome of body shame or the obsessive self-consciousness stealing our confidence in all areas of life.[5]

We constantly worry: are we thin enough, muscular enough, or pretty enough?

I hope you and I agree: enough is enough.

A body image spray-painted with shame manifests in several ways, such as extreme unhappiness about how we look, distorted self-perception (i.e., we believe we're bigger or smaller than reality and feel unsure about how we look to others), harsh attitudes and language toward our bodies, excessive body checking (i.e., tugging, pulling, or pinching parts), and thoughts about how we look dominating our minds.

There's a difference between acknowledging a flaw and obsessing over one. It's one thing to acknowledge a feature you wished were better on occasion. It's another thing to be significantly dissatisfied to the point of feeling shame, hatred, and contempt for how you look.

Is this you?

Body shame sounds like this:

- I hate my stomach!
- I'd be a fox if I didn't have this big butt.
- I can't go sleeveless. Have you seen my arms?
- My nose ruins my whole face. I need a nose job.
- My thighs can light a fire they're so thick.
- I have chicken legs. I can't wear shorts.
- I can't be seen bald. Where's my toupee?
- Do I look fat?

How many criticisms do you have about your body each day? A Whole & Free Health course participant admitted to twenty-one times that she had to stop her thoughts from criticizing her body within one day. Imagine your boss giving you twenty-one criticisms about your work each day. Would you want to work for that person?

Probably not. You'd quit, switch departments, or get promoted. Unlike your boss, your body isn't fire-able. You're the boss of your body. You can't escape your body. You can't move from it. And you certainly can't switch it for someone else's.

Since your body and soul is an until-death-do-you-part relationship, you might as well learn how to enjoy and care for it.

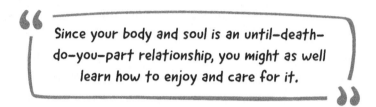

Since your body and soul is an until-death-do-you-part relationship, you might as well learn how to enjoy and care for it.

Body Image Facts

About 90 percent of us have some area of negativity around our bodies.[6] The problem isn't wishing your nose was smaller or lips were bigger. It's having a strong preoccupation about how we look that negatively impacts life, work, relationships, eating behaviors, and food choices.

Psychology Today partnered with eating disorder director Dr. David Garner, PhD, to find insights into body image health factors by performing a study of 3,453 women and 548 men in a famous Body Image Survey.[7]

Fifty-six percent of women were unhappy about their overall appearance with most dissatisfaction about the belly, weight, and backside.[8] Whereas 43 percent of men were unhappy with their overall appearance with most dissatisfaction about the belly, weight, muscle definition, and chest.[9]

Take a look at the Body Worry Chart. Which body parts upset you the most?

our obsessions
BODY PARTS WE WORRY ABOUT MOST

MEN		WOMEN

3   average number **of body parts** we worry about   6

MEN	body part	WOMEN
17%	natural hair	32%
21%	gray hair	29%
24%	thinning hair	18%
20%	facial hair	27%
10%	eyebrows	22%
9%	nose	10%
4%	lips	8%
11%	wrinkles	28%
23%	skin	40%
10%	chin/neck	27%
8%	arms	23%
7%	hands	13%
9%	nails	18%
15%	excess body hair	15%
14%	chest/breasts	24%
52%	stomach	69%
5%	cellulite	29%
7%	butt	29%
4%	hips	25%
5%	thighs	36%
5%	legs	20%
2%	ankles	5%
8%	feet	12%

67% of adult women worry about their appearance regularly - more often than finances, health, relationships or professional success

Illustration 26.1   Body Worry Chart[10]

Sixty percent of body dissatisfaction came from body weight.[11] But the study proved that the more unhappy with our body we are, then the more we'll struggle with a higher body mass index. Those who were fifty or more pounds from their ideal weight struggled with body image the most versus those within a five-pound range who struggled the least. [12]

Not surprisingly, most women wanted to lose body fat, but men wanted to gain muscle.

The struggle with body image begins early. Fifty to 80 percent of young women and 25 percent of young men start to feel dissatisfied with their bodies as teens and even pre-teens.[13]

Like adults, young men want toned and defined muscles, whereas young women want thinness. And 81 percent of young women fear fatness which causes weight problems, strengthening the shame-diet-binge-weight gain cycle.[14]

In a study of 1,196 teenage girls, researchers found that the ones who weren't concerned about their weight and had a positive outlook about their bodies fared well with their weight well into adulthood.[15]

However, 59 percent of those who thought negatively about their weight and bodies, despite a normal weight, ended up becoming overweight or obese in adulthood.[16] So the proof is in the pudgy beliefs per Chapter 17. The fear of fatness or self-perception of fatness usually leads to more, not less, fatness.

Body image concerns are growing amongst youth, leading to sad projections in areas of mental, emotional, physical, and spiritual health.

Where Does Body Image Come From?

The media is the top source of body shame thoughts for all of us. Fifty-seven percent of women feel more insecure after engaging with social media or watching television.[17] We cannot help but compare ourselves at times to those who make it to the big screen or the social scene.

Media is a large part of the problem. Seeing underweight women, extra buff men, and food porn commercials makes for our severe discontentment with our bodies. Since the big screen is so difficult to get on, actors, actresses, athletes, news anchors, and others are naturally assigned more value because they are the one percent of society who get to be seen by everyone. And those one-percenters look far more glorious than the rest of us toads (in our minds) because they've made it.

Then we watch, comparing ourselves to the finely sculpted echelons of society, get depressed because we don't measure up, see a commercial for cheesy bread, order it, and sulk in our feelings of fatness.

Watch, eat, sulk, repeat.

Reduce visual media (television, internet, magazines, and social) and you'll get an immediate boost in self-esteem.

The sulking in fatness and food temptations leads to poor body stewardship, which is the next major source of body shame. You know this from Chapters 7–12. If we exercise, eat well, and sleep well, we'll increase a positive body image. Those who exercise report increased self-esteem, confidence, and positive feelings about their bodies.[18]

We drop weighty guilt when we do the things that we know we should do like drink water instead of pop, get rest instead of staying up late, and take a walk instead of sitting on the couch. We also know our problem foods create a downward emotional spiral with a not-so-fabulous pity party for our body image sentiment.

Youth are battered by media from an early age to perceive lean as worthy of love and value. Studies show nearly 66 percent of television shows and movies portray lean men and underweight women to have positive traits such as love and joy, while 75 percent of television shows and movies associate those who are heavier with negative traits such as sadness, aggressive attitudes, or laziness.[19] This further supports weight biases and body image dissatisfaction.

A non-media source of body image formation are words spoken about your body. Negative words spoken to us like Sheila received, "You have horse lips!" or Frank received, "You're a double wide taking up the whole street" promote body shame.

Word attacks on our bodies from other adults or kids stick with us as does a lack of affirming words about our bodies from parents, peers, or siblings. And if we don't have positive references about our bodies, we'll fail to see our bodies as positive aspects of who we are.

If the negative words are spoken from a love interest that's especially brutal on our body image because another major non-media source of body image is how our love interest makes us feel about our bodies and what they say. We feel special when someone we love thinks we have a beautiful smile or nice backside. We seek out positive body opinions of the one who gets to touch us intimately. Lord knows we all secretly wish to be worshipped for our sexy bodies by our spouses even if we're not so sexy or spouse-less at the moment.

Criticism from our love interest deeply damages self-esteem, like Marie whose husband made snide comments about what she ate and wore or George whose wife refused to be intimate with him because of his size.

Fat jokes or constant requests to lose weight from our loved ones, especially a spouse, require clear boundaries and a desire to change for oneself, not anyone else.

Lastly, we learn from our parents. If our father or mother shamed his or her body, we more than likely will shame ours. At least 80 percent of children of parents who have eating disorders will also have one, and the same is true for body shame.[20]

Children by nature adopt their belief systems from their parents. If a child sees his or her parents dieting or professing that they're not thin enough, the child will gather his or her self-worth from those things the parent approves of, such as thinness.

In other words, body shame like obesity usually transfers from generation to generation if not overcome. We'll work on undoing the damages done in Part Two.

Looks'ology: Psychological Roots of Body Image

I've seen several clients in my therapy practice who've performed daily self-floggings in their critical attitudes toward their body, and I've found that there are psychological, spiritual causes as well. I call these psychological roots of body image, Looks'ology.

Looks'ology
(Looks-o-lo-gee)
is the made-up, psychological name for why we use
looks to distract us from maturing spiritually and emotionally

Masked Negative Emotions

Masked negative emotions can affect how we feel about body parts. An obsession on a body part can divert our attention from negative emotions happening in deeper areas of life.

In other words, we mask negative emotions by focusing on physical criticism or by the over attention to looking good.

Elle chronically picked at her acne and obsessed with the flaws of her face in the mirror. After we dug deeper, she found her impulsive body shaming masked her deep insecurity of not knowing who she was and what she was to do with her life.

As a twenty something, she was dependent on her parents and afraid to grow up. After addressing these fears in therapy practice, her chronic body (face) shaming disappeared, and she resolved her deep insecurities about her future and her abilities to face it.

Look for ways that you're overcritical of an outward body part when you're upset with something else. Emotional Fitness practices can help you to get to the heart of your negative body criticism. Do the actions in chapter for emotional fitness.

Ungratefulness

We have an extreme lack of gratitude with our Creator's make of us. Ungratefulness has its roots in covetousness or jealousy. We want more and are unhappy with what we have.

Gia was a healthy weight. She worked out often, ate well, and was filled with the Holy Spirit, but she was plagued with body shame in her mind. Despite being a small size, she insisted that she was heavy and obsessed with cellulite and other features of her body that she deemed unattractive.

Her body shame was most pronounced on an island vacation. Each time she went to the pool, her thoughts slung whips at her body, making harsh comparisons to every other women's body shape. And she felt the chronic insecurity that theirs was better than hers despite her beautiful, lean, and healthy body.

When someone was bigger, she felt superior.

Often, Gia pinched at her thighs and condemned herself for cellulite, thinking everyone was thinking about it too. In her frustration, sometimes she'd punch the body parts she hated.

Gia's low self-esteem was projected onto her body. Instead of feeling worthy of peace and freedom from body shame, the shame kept her bound in her thoughts.

Let's be thankful and content in all things, including when we feel inadequate, insecure, or jealous,

Self-Rejection

We can reject ourselves and our appearance because we may not know, like, and trust who we are. Sharon hated her nose so much that she declined socializing opportunities because of fear of others looking at her. She couldn't be herself since her obsession with her schnozzle took the time that would otherwise be used to get to know herself and others.

Our body is a beautiful expression of God's design of us and our ancestry. Our looks magnify the beauty of the family members who have gone before us. To reject a part of us is also to reject some aspect of who we are.

Unworthiness

Unworthiness shows up as vanity or neglect of our looks and appearance altogether. We can attempt to cover our low self-worth with expensive name brand clothing or material things, an over-attention to appearance (excessive mirror time), or excessive makeup.

Vanity is a stronghold of believing self-worth is how we look and causes us to strive for false ideologies of beauty perfection. Unworthiness is deep in one's soul that manifests as a cause of shame, including body shame and weight and eating bondage.

The other side of unworthiness is poor hygiene and dingy, ripped, or ill-fitting clothing. Unworthiness is healed best by crying out to God and allowing His soul surgery to heal it. It's not healed with more makeup, calf implants, or longer workouts.

Looks'ology helps us to see beyond the distraction of hating our looks to find spiritual and psychological roots for wholeness and freedom.

And sometimes the deficit of truth extends body shame into a class of its own—body dysmorphia disorder.

An Introduction to Body Dysmorphic Disorder (BDD)

If you suspect your body image concerns are extreme, you're not alone. In the United States about 2.5 percent of females and 2.2 percent of males have body dysmorphic disorder (BDD).[21]

Abused and neglected individuals develop BDD at a higher rate, making past childhood-trauma a considerable risk factor along with genetic and physiological predispositions.

Body Dysmorphia Disorder Examples

Once I saw at the gym who needed to get to Kentucky Fried Chicken ASAP. Many anorexics couldn't be that way unless there was a true perception of their body image that was distorted. They think they're fat, and the image in their head is believed more than the actual image in the mirror.

In the same way it's possible for an obese person to have a perception of thinness in their minds. Any mental body image distortion will cause eating portion distortion—too little food like in the case of anorexic or too much food as in the case for morbid obesity.

In a simple Google search, you can see how body dysmorphia disorder and the spirit of vanity caused good looking folks to become unnatural looking with plastic surgery.

For example, Pixie Fox had ribs removed to reduce her waist and at least seventeen surgeries and counting to look like a Barbie doll.[22] And Rodrigo Alves' search for perfection caused him to pursue at least forty-seven surgeries to become the human Ken doll. He has since decided to become a woman and changed his name to Jessica.[23,24]

And you that thought you had problems.

I wish medicine were holistic with mental, emotional, and spiritual health treatment as this kind of drive for beauty is a supreme health risk, a call for deliverance, and a clear mental health matter.

Body Dysmorphic Disorder Check [25]

YES (X)	BODY DYSMORPHIC DISORDER (BDD) CRITERION
	Do you have a preoccupation with one or more perceived defects in physical appearance that are not observable or appear slight to others?
	At some point during the course of the disorder, do you experience repetitive skin picking, mirror checking, excessive grooming, and other things?
	Do the behaviors or thoughts cause distress or impairment in occupational, social, or other important areas of functioning?
	Do you have constant concern about your appearance?

Muscle Dysmorphia Check [26]

YES (X)	MUSCLE DYSMORPHIA CRITERION
	Do you meet the Body Dysmorphic Disorder Criterion?
	Do you have concerns that your muscle build is insufficient?

Important: This check is not a diagnosis. Please see a professional for help if you believe you have body dysmorphic disorder for a full evaluation and treatment plan.

BDD is a form of obsessive-compulsive disorder and has a high suicidal rate and risk in those who suffer from it. If you suspect you have an obsession or a distorted image of yourself, please seek professional help today. I've observed those who continually gorge with food and fatten their bodies have a deep form of BDD.

God, The Master Artist

BDD and body shame hijack God's messages about our bodies. If we don't change this relationship we have with our bodies, we'll be in a never-ending Weight & Eating War.

Let's jump off the body shame train.

How To Jump Off the Body Shame Train for Good!

To get off the body shame train we'll need a one-way ticket to God-fidence. We may not be the happiest about how we look today, but as we embrace body honor and heal shame, we're sure to be happier with who we are and how we look in times to come.

We have a big giant to defeat, so we'll use several strategies to do so. Let's get started.

Receive Your Uniqueness

Why is it that when we're born into the world, people rub our bums and think we're the most perfect little thing ever. Then we grow up, and we think that we're the worst-looking troll on this side of heaven?

The first stop on the body shame train is to make your only standard of beauty God's standard.

When our definition of our beauty aligns with God's definition, we can heal distorted body shame. His definition is that what He has made is very good, good-looking, and good enough.

Here's the thing: when you're the only one, rare creation that you are, you are perfect immeasurable beauty. The onslaught of media and cultural ideals for beauty cause us to forget the fact that we're divine expressions of our beautiful God.

Yes, you forgot that you're the only one of you created by God.

> " When you're the only one, rare creation that you are, you are perfect immeasurable beauty. The onslaught of media and cultural ideals for beauty cause us to forget. "

There's no one else on our planet of over 7 billion people or in the entire galaxy like you. No one else is you. No one else has your history, experiences, interests, personality, talents, and skills in the exact make up like you. And no one has the exact same body chemistry, fingerprints, hair, voice, or face.

We look at our scars and imperfections and think, *I'm so fat and ugly.* But when you don't feel attractive, you use some basis to judge because how do you know that you're not attractive?

Ask yourself in who's opinion am I not attractive? And if it's your opinion, then ask yourself by what standards? You'll find that you're measuring yourself based on standards unconsciously set for you.

The worlds standards haven't changed much. Worldly standards are about 48 pounds lighter and 6 inches taller than the average women who is 5'4 and nearly 171 pounds as of 2018.[29] And a chest size of 5 inches smaller, biceps of 3 inches smaller, and a waistline of 11 inches smaller than the average male who is 5'9, 199 pounds, and has a 40-inch waist respectively.[30]

The world judges on skin color, ethnicity, height, symmetrical features, hair, body size, chest size (for men and women), skin clarity, and arm size, but who set these standards?

Even experts say our standards of beauty are arbitrary.

Martha Beck said, "Although beauty may be in the eye of the beholder, the feeling of being beautiful exists solely in the mind of the beheld. Standards of beauty are arbitrary. Body shame exists only to the extent that our physiques don't match our own beliefs about how we should look. Good-looking individuals are treated better than homely ones in virtually every social situation, from dating to trial by jury."[31]

She says we mostly measure against our own ideals of beauty. So, we need to shake up those ideals within our minds and from media.

Look at the magazine cover example with Faith Hill. Notice how much thinner her back, arm, and face are in the promoted cover versus her photo.

WHAT IMAGE ARE YOU LIVING UP TO

Image 26.2 Cover photo shop example[32]

If you or the world sets standards for how you should look, then you'll never measure up. The world's standard is photoshopped and artificially contrived—also known as a lie. And there we go again listening to the lies and rejecting the truth that what God made is very good.

Since He is the Creator of all people, He also gets to create the standard. And because you are whole, unique, and complete all on your own, definition of single defined by Dr. Miles Monroe, you are one of a kind.[33]

Something one of a kind is immeasurable because the only thing to measure against is itself.

That means whatever your size or shape doesn't matter.

Your beauty is a nonnegotiable truth of Creation.

There's only one standard, and it's *whatever you are.* Your eyes, your nose, your hair, your bone structure is perfect. Like an oak tree, a red rose, the North Star, or a snowflake are perfect, so are you. Appreciate all your nooks, crannies, life-lived, and other unique attributes that make you—you.

> There's only one standard, and it's whatever you are.

You are beautiful. You are handsome. Are you willing to stop the world's standards? Will you accept your body and looks as His gifts to you? And accept your looks are your gift to others? Yes, your perfectly imperfect package is a beautifully wrapped gift to others too.

> Appreciate all your nooks, crannies, life-lived, and other unique attributes that make you—you.

Are you willing to let go of your own standards for ideal beauty?

From now on receive your God-given uniqueness and accept that the only true standard of beauty is God's. Repeat after me, "I receive my uniqueness and beauty. Thank you for every part of how you made me."

Live the Body Honor Manifesto

Our next stop is the body honor manifesto because the opposite of body shame is body honor. Each principle is also a strategy as well. Repeat the following confessions often to heal body shame.

The Body Honor Manifesto – 9 Principles To Increase Body Respect, Love, and Confidence

Principle #1 – Talk kindly. "I only talk kindly to my body."

If we're kind to our body, it will be all the more kind in return. When we offer compassion to our insecurities, our emotional body feels safe to release all that's unwanted from our lives, including unsupportive mindsets, people, weight, and habits.

Kindness kills criticism.

Kindness is like honey that is sweet to the soul and brings healing to our bones (Proverbs 16:24). Proverbs 18:20 tells us that the power of life or death is in the tongue.

> " Kindness kills criticism. "

Words thought and spoken to us have power in shaping our body image.

Body image is largely formed as a child. In one study among female students, 80 percent of them claimed that their body shame started with negative remarks made by friends and family.[34] And 73 percent of women and 57 percent of men believed their negative body thoughts began from being teased.[35]

We're soul's inside of our human body, and we only know what we look like based on people's comments and our own image in the mirror, especially as small children. By nature we listen to what others say about how we look; therefore, to heal we need to consider not only our own thoughts but also what others have said about our looks.

EXERCISE: HEALING THE UNKIND

QUIZ

Step 1: Make a list of all the negative things told to you about your body and that you've thought about your body. List your approximate age at the time.

Here are a few examples that contributed to my body shame:

Age 7: "You're getting fat." (my grandmother; I was far from fat)

Age 8: "You're so boney! Get off my lap." (my aunt)

Age 9: "You're skin and bones, I'm calling you Twiggy!" (my grandfather)

Ages 10–12: "Twiggy!" (my grandfather, when referring to me countless times with roaring laughter)

Age 13: "You need to lose some weight to be a model with us." (a modeling school)

Age 13: "You jolly green giant." (a popular peer in my class; you know how that ended)

Age 14: "You're spreading." (my grandmother, right in front of my boyfriend)

Age 15: "Nothing looks good on me. I wish I was skinnier." (me, getting ready for a school dance). The shaming of others now internalized.

Step 2: One by one, share those negative thoughts and comments with the Lord in prayer. Ask the Holy Spirit to heal you from the lies about your body. Simple prayers like: "God, I ask you to remove every hurt and damage done when I was called Twiggy. Heal me, Father."

Step 3: Repent to God for the critical words, thoughts, and treatments you've done toward your body. Also apologize to your body by saying, "I'm so sorry, body, for treating you harshly and saying that you're ugly and unhealthy."

Step 4: Make a list of all the positive things said and thought about your body/looks.

Step 5: Go to a bathroom mirror and look at yourself. Start with saying, "I love you," in the mirror to begin to build a stronger relationship with yourself and your body. Ask God for help to see you as He sees you.

In a study by *Hope College*, it was concluded that those who repeat Scriptures over themselves have an improved sense of body confidence.[36] So, speak Psalm 139:13–14 over yourself and other Scriptures that resonate. Then, for every negative thing on your list, speak something positive over yourself.

How would your body image have been different if affirming words were spoken? Every time you look in a mirror speak truth and affirm yourself. Do this Healing the Unkind exercise to heal body shame any time. Talk often to your body to build a positive, strong relationship with it.

Principle #2 – Thank it. "I'm thankful for my body."

A woman asked me, "What is it you're doing to lose weight?"

My response, "Being grateful."

In my early attempts at weight loss, even when I achieved the target weight, I was ungrateful evidenced by obsessing over my body's imperfections. Oftentimes we look at old photos and wish we would've appreciated ourselves more at the smaller size, am I right?

As discussed, gratitude with our body is also gratitude to God. Gratitude is also an amazing antidote for body shame because gratitude opens the gates of heaven and draws us nearer to God (Psalm 100:4).

Choose to be thankful for the outside and the inside of you.

Don't just see your eyes looking around doing their thing. See that your eyes see the beauty of your grandmother's smile or daughter's joy. Your heart pumps blood all day every day. And your intestines stretch their digestive muscles with every meal.

Thank your body for all its hard work.

Thank God for every part of the body and what that part allows you to have in your life. I walk you through this in *The Body Love Prayer* in Non-Edible Goodies. That prayer did wonders for me to heal my distorted body image and increase my gratitude for it. Keep a simple practice of thanking God for each part as you bathe or dress.

Principle #3 – Accept it. "I accept my body as it is."

Dana Christmas had beautiful skin, a smile that lit up the room, bright eyes, and stylish haircuts. Twenty-four hours later she was unrecognizable. She had severe second and third degree burns on 60 percent of her body, including her head and face.[37]

A horrific fire at my university killed three students and injured fifty-eight people.[38] As a resident assistant, she was burned in her heroic attempt to rescue other dorm students from the greedy flames. In one crazy night all that mattered was that she was alive. Nothing else was important—not her weight, her looks, her hair, or her hand that was deformed because of the fire. This puts things into perspective, doesn't it?

Do her scars of heroism make her any less beautiful? No, because her scars show the beauty of who she is and what she did to help so many others.

We can stop self-rejection when we get our perspectives straight.

Somewhere in the world someone wishes to have a body or features like yours. People are dying right now who can only dream of another chance to better treat their bodies to see their legacy.

Reflections on perspective help stir acceptance. It feels counterintuitive to appreciate your body when you've gained significant weight. But the weight gained could be double or triple in today's food addictive culture.

It really could be worse.

When you feel rejected, unappreciative, demanding, or harsh toward your body and its features, take a moment to reflect on how much worse it could be to cultivate more acceptance of your current appearance.

Principle #4 – Enjoy it. "I enjoy life in my body."

Enjoyment is an extension of our gratitude by practicing active acknowledgement and appreciation for our body as a companion. You're in partnership with it. And you want to enjoy the work you do in it. Cleaning, driving, walking, sitting—all of it can be done with enjoyment.

It's like that house with no paintings on the walls. When we hang up the artwork, it's a sign we've settled in, that we're making a home a home. How can you settle into your body? What can you do to be at home in it?

To enjoy your body is also to take some healthy pride in your appearance. Your clothes express your personality. But sometimes body shame can make us wear boring, revealing, baggy, or black clothing all the time.

So, for the love of God and all things beautiful, don't wear so much black. I do think the grief of body shame shows up in enormous amounts of dark clothing, especially black to look slim.

Your body's like, "Geez, another funeral today."

Help it out.

Dress in a way that brings out your joy. Try out new styles or colors and adjust the fit to get the size right. Match your clothes to match the Whole & Free you, not the old broken and bound version. Could you use a makeover?

 Match your clothes to match the Whole & Free you, not the old broken and bound version.

We feel enjoyment when we take time for adventure, workouts, or sports to get our hearts pumping and muscles moving. We're meant to live. We feel alive as we express physical energy. Brenda felt every part of her body when she went ziplining at age sixty! And Carolyn took on running and ran a half marathon at forty-three. How can you experience more life in your body?

To practice enjoyment is also to be present in your body. Those who have experienced physical or sexual abuse may have trouble being in their bodies. They dissociate from it. To dissociate is to disconnect from feeling grounded and connected to your body.

If you feel like you're out-of-body at times or floating, check out *The Body Keeps the Score* by psychiatrist Bessel A. van der Kolk to heal any post-traumatic stress disorder (PTSD) to better enjoy life in your body.[39]

Principle #5 – Trust it. "I trust my body."

A relationship of trust is the foundation for any positive relationship. Do you trust your body? Have you felt betrayed by it?

We've had to rely on our bodies to act right when giving birth or climbing a ladder.

Incidents we've had when our bodies seemingly failed us, like a birth going wrong or a back going out, can feel like betrayal to us, not to mention when we've experienced abuse, injuries, sickness, disabilities, or accidents.

Yet the body gives frequent signs that something is off nutritionally, emotionally, or spiritually in our lives. For many of the physical ailments and injuries we attract in life, there are emotional reasons too.

 The body gives frequent signs that something is off nutritionally, emotionally, or spiritually in our lives.

Somatization is the technical term for when we manifest health concerns due to unresolved emotional issues. When in chronic pain, we need to also route out the soul pain as even chronic pain has a higher resolution success rate when we deal with past trauma and get psychotherapy.

So, we can trust when the body isn't working properly. It's using pain or the experience to tell us something about how our inputs nutritionally, emotionally, or spiritually need attention.

Reflect on your trust or mistrust in your relationship with your body. Do you trust your body? How can you trust it more?

Principle #6 – Listen to it. "I listen to my body."

Intuitively we know what our bodies need if we take a moment to listen. How well do you listen to what your body is saying?

As we hear and obey the body's still small voice, we can trust that it's leading us to a better wellbeing. It whispers, "Sleep," "Water," "Move,"

"Stand up," "Eat light," or "Please, don't eat cheese; you know how much it hurts me."

As you might recall from, the flesh is our soul's use of the body to carry out its carnal desires for self-harm and indulgence. The body is a miraculous sensory vessel and carries out the soul's will and or God's will.

Your body seeks to be attuned to your soul.

The body and the flesh have different voices.

Your physical body speaks like your soul speaks, only it requests the most basic needs. Intuitively we can hear what we're to eat, drink, and do, but it's difficult to hear when we have a Standard American Diet manipulating it.

But the mind can be conflicted because both brain and taste buds can be manipulated with highly palatable foods. But because the body is scientific in nature, it always seeks your highest good.

Our body doesn't ever want chemicalized non-foods or sugar, fat, and salt-laden foods. It doesn't ask for them. Therefore, it's important to hear beyond your emotional body—and even your beast's addictive voice—to hear the true voice of the body.

It takes practice to hear, but you can learn its voice and intuitively eat your way to better health. As I cleaned up my Standard American Diet, I heard it more clearly.

Pauline decided to listen after a binge episode. She found that her body needed a balanced meal and rest instead of taking on more projects. She wanted to bulldoze past her physical needs, but not listening triggered bingeing.

Amber complained for months about her exhaustion. After taking a few moments to listen to her body's needs, she knew that she needed to stop her protein bars and eat real food. She also figured that electronics at night stole sleep quality. So, she put her phone in another room to charge and focused on an earlier bedtime to honor her body's voice properly.

Check in with your body more often. As we listen to its requests, a beautiful relationship with it emerges that will manifest more body, soul, and spirit freedom in our lives.

Principle #7 – Heal it. "I heal my body."

Imagine that you were taking a shower, and before you could finish cleaning up, mud was thrown on you. So, you started the water again to get the mud off, only it happened repeatedly, which made it difficult to get cleaned up so that you can go to relax. After some time, a guard went up around the shower to protect you from the mud splash so that you can finally get to relax.

Well, the body is turning on the shower itself. It's constantly looking for what's out of order or doesn't belong. It utilizes a sophisticated system to get to its highest degree of health.

The water is the right habits—eating well, exercising, and so on that support the natural cleansing process of the body to heal itself.

The mud is all that doesn't serve you. It's the Standard American Diet and lifestyle we're engaged in daily that prevents us from healing.

The guard is the boundaries you need to put in place to protect your body from unnecessary harm—physically, emotionally, and spiritually.

The Body H.A.B.I.T.S. have a direct impact on a positive body image and heal your body. Hydration (H) reduces negative feelings and bloating. Activity (A) directly boosts body positivity immediately after exercising.[40] Move your body to remove body shame.

Balancing (B) hormones helps because 75 percent of women feel body shame around their cycles due to water retention and less active happy chemicals in the body.[41] Nutrient Loading (I) pours love into our minds and cells. Detoxing (T) gets unloving stuff out of them. And sleep (S) boosts happy brain chemicals and weight reduction.

Apply tips for implementing the Body H.A.B.I.T.S. in your life. (Reference Chapters 7–12.)

Principle #8 – Look at it. "I look at myself with appreciation."

Validate a healthy body image by looking at yourself. In the thick of my disorder, I couldn't look in the mirror. I looked down when looking at other humans. Body haters have a difficult time looking in the mirror without a slew of thoughts about how upset they feel about their image staring back.

If I passed a mirror in office buildings, stores, or hallways, I'd scurry quickly by it. I piled on my makeup to protect others from seeing the ugly I felt inside.

Do the opposite.

Smile at yourself when you walk past the mirror. Stop the "oh no, don't take a photo" drama when someone wants to snap a shot. Don't pretend your body isn't there or doesn't matter, hide when there's a video camera, or allow your body shame to hold you back from sharing your message on social media.

Expose the shame.

For some of us it would be the most horrendous thing to wear a bathing suit in the open. A lady pastor posted herself in a revealing bathing suit on Facebook. At first, I judged the immodesty, but she shared about her body shame that had plagued her throughout her life. Her post helped her to get free of body shame. Despite anyone else's negative judgment, she healed her own. Most cheered her on to support her liberation.

Sometimes we need to expose the shame for it to heal. For me, I felt my thighs were too fat to wear shorts for a long time. To heal I had to start wearing shorts with confidence. It helped to have a friend take a photo of me in shorts so that I could see that shorts looked fine. No one noticed or cared about the flaws I saw.

You know people are too worried about their own big butt to worry about yours. Several clients were afraid to go sleeveless because of flapping arm fat, but to hide in shame is to wear a long-sleeved shirt in the middle of blazing summer heat.

It doesn't make sense.

Wear the sleeveless shirt and expose the shame. So what, a flapping arm in the wind never hurt anybody. Embracing flawed parts gets the shame out. Shame loves hiding and covering up. So, be sure to talk about your body shame with your accountability partner or a friend like I did with my shorts issue.

Once exposed, shame has no more power.

Show parts of your body that you've hidden due to body shame. To continue to heal the shame take great care of yourself too. Sixty percent of people felt their body shame was due to excess weight.[42] We need to both accept where we are and actively pursue prosperous health and freedom.

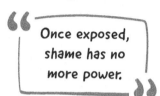

> Once exposed, shame has no more power.

Also, just because we can wear something, doesn't mean we should. Modesty is a virtue, and even though we have admirable parts, it's a virtue to not to have to show them off. So, be mindful because pride puffs up as much as shame hides.

Principle #9 – Love it. "My body is sacred and special. I love it."

Do you feel your body is sacred? Holy? Special? How do you treat something precious? Do you nurture it? Do you take special care?

We're vessels of the wine of the Spirit. We're filled with the love, peace, and the power of God.

Let's grow out of the body shame-based dieting, workout forcing, and body manipulation to embrace our sacredness, specialness, and preciousness.

Let's work the Body H.A.B.I.T.S. from a motive of divine love and wisdom for our sacredness, not worldly harshness to force the body into change.

As we learn to love our bodies, we'll value them as vessels of the souls and spirits they hold within them.

Have you ever broken a glass with your favorite beverage in it? We're upset that we didn't get to enjoy the beverage. We value the container because we value what's in it. Your container, your body, is so precious. Treat it like it is.

Eat like you love yourself too.

Standard American Diet fare has no love in it. It doesn't heal the body. It steals from the body and mind. Because these foods are built on profit and taste motives only, when we eat them, we're sowing this all-take-rude nature into our bodies as well. These foods harvest shame—body shame.

We reap what we sow. Sow love into your body with what you eat and how you care for it. Food made with light and love give light and love to the body and mind as well.

> **Food made with light and love give light and love to the body and mind as well.**

End Comparisons

Bonita, a talented, successful career woman struggled with raging comparisons of her body with everyone else's bodies. She thought, *I'm not as fit as Christy, or I look much slimmer than Pat.*

Body comparison is a source of pain because it's rooted in you feeling insufficient or superior.

This jealousy is a constant inner thought war of how we're perceived by others or look in comparison to others, possibly causing disorder in how we eat.

Bonita wouldn't have been able to move forward to emotional wholeness or freedom if she didn't admit that she was harassed by comparisons.

I took Bonita to the mirror.

She looked into her own eyes. I guided as she spoke acceptance to each part of her physical appearance and thanked it for what that part did for her and how the body part made her special.

Mirror work is the fastest way I've seen my clients grow in self-acceptance.

Do the same. Go to the mirror, look into your eyes, and speak the truth. Do the mirror work to validate yourself and let go of comparing and judging others in their bodies.

Claim inside your mind, *I am beautiful and so are you* to others. While you're at it say, "I have a beautiful body." Each man and woman is is or her own beautiful.

And our own beliefs we hold about our looks impact body shame the most. It's important to believe that you're good looking enough and your body is beautiful enough. Even on your worse hair day, validate your body with thoughts like *I am beautiful* and *I am beautiful no matter how I look at the moment.*

Another way to stop comparing is to give and receive compliments. Receive compliments well by saying a simple thank you. And please don't follow up a compliment with how bad your skin looks or how little you paid for your outfit.

When tempted to feel jealous or superior, share an encouragement with the one you want to compare. Be generous with kind words by giving compliments more. When you think a kind word about someone, tell them.

No more hater'ade against your body or anyone else's body.

Magnify Your Soul's Qualities

What if you took the energy focused on the body's flaws and put it toward growing your character? To magnify your soul's qualities is to value who you are more than your looks.

When we acknowledge our accomplishments and who we are, we can heal body shame. Keisha's body shame reduced when she acknowledged that she was a loving spouse and mother. She also celebrated that she started a company, was an incredible swimmer, saved her money well, and gave birth.

As we value our life's meaning, our character, and soul qualities, we'll reduce the power of our looks as the sole measurement of self-worth. And we'll be more confident in our bodies. In other words, we'll focus less on the zit and more on the beauty of the whole face. We need to

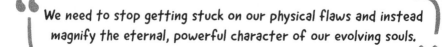

We need to stop getting stuck on our physical flaws and instead magnify the eternal, powerful character of our evolving souls.

stop getting stuck on our physical flaws and instead magnify the eternal, powerful character of our evolving souls. Make a list of all of your soul's qualities, accomplishments, and character strengths.

What do you value about who you are? What accomplishments in your life support your confidence? What other areas of life can support more meaning?

Reduce Media

Media says, "You're too big, so buy this diet pill." But the Body H.A.B.I.T.S. will lead you to your natural size. Or "You're hungry for dinner, you need this bacon cheeseburger with secret sauce," when you have an honest meal in the fridge.

Media impacts distortion and depression around our bodies and food behaviors. Eighty percent of women admit that watching television makes them feel insecure.[43]

Media shows women who are slightly underweight. The average Victoria Secrets fashion model is a size 4, while the average size of women is U.S. is size 14.[44] Female models are 5'10" and 114 pounds (and probably a tween!) on average.[45] Male models are 6'0" and 167 on average.[46]

As a culture, we watch an insane amount of television and movies and consume a great deal of social media. We create an ideal image to compare ourselves to. The problem is that we don't, and we won't, ever measure up. The standard or bar is too high, which creates a constant sense of failure and low self-esteem.

Instead of trying, let go—not of your body care but of media and the constant self-berating, apologizing, and isolating because of body shame against an ideal that isn't possible except by manipulation of images. Reduce social media, television, and movie watching, and body-esteem will increase.

Pay attention to your body shame feelings after engaging with media to see how it affects you. How much television and social media do you watch? How can you reduce this to support a positive body image?

Adjust Your Lenses

Noemi, a beautiful Mexican mother and grandmother, struggled her whole life with her body image. She was made fun of for her weight and her face by peers and loved ones. She was told to wear her hair long to cover up her "ugly face."

After much turmoil, she decided to talk to God about it. She prayed, "Lord, help me to see me like You see me."

And she saw a vision of herself happy with short hair. She saw herself for the first time as Spirit saw her, and she wept.

She was beautiful. Everything else she believed was a lie.

She cut her hair and felt joy about her looks.

Take note that the best counselor on body shame is the Holy Spirit. He can give you new eyes.

Have you been a healthy weight but still see yourself in your mind's eye at your heaviest weight? Or you can't seem to shake the fat girl or boy image inside?

Sherry in the Whole & Free Health course was an athlete in high school. Back then, she was able to eat whatever she wanted and didn't gain a pound. Fast forward twenty years ... she ate the same, but she saw herself as a teenage athlete. Her body image distortion saw herself as thinner than reality.

We can do the following to adjust our body image goggles:

- Look in the mirror (say something kind while you're there)
- Weigh yourself (limit to once per week, day, or month)
- Take measurements and date them
- Compare past and present images of yourself to gauge how you felt about your body at the time of the photos
- Take exercise classes so that you can see yourself amongst other people in the mirrors to get a better handle on your body size
- Take consistent action to create a healthier body, soul, and spirit

These steps help to focus on internal self-image to the external reality. As we work on our body honor, God will adjust our lens.

Take Action

Gather images of yourself from the past and reflect on how you felt about yourself. Were you happy with yourself, or were you still feeling insecure about your body shape and size?

Final Destination: Welcome to God'fidence!

You can change how you eat, your clothing style, your workouts, and your body composition. But body image is in a hard-to-reach box in the crevasse of the attic, and it's difficult to get in there and clean it out. It's a heavy box too.

So, it requires some help to get it out of there and into the trash.

For me, body shame took a tremendous amount of prayer, which is always our fundamental defense in everything. I was plagued with body shame at my smallest and certainly at my heaviest. Prayer delivered dreams (night) to help me heal as well as my practicing all these strategies. Other clients and students also had miraculous healings as well.

One last thing: our self-image is our beliefs about how we see ourselves in our own minds, and it also needs to adjust with our body image. We can't continue to see ourselves as lazy, unhealthy, fat, addicted, and tired.

How we see ourselves limits or expands our biggest dreams for our lives.

> How we see ourselves limits or expands our biggest dreams for our lives.

You must embrace the transition from the old version of yourself, including the "insecure, heavier" you, to the new "secure, lighter" version of yourself. Otherwise, we will regain back up to the image that we believe we are.

We act in direct accordance with who we believe we are. If you believe your unattractive and don't have value, you'll demonstrate that through actions of self-harm like promiscuity, or desperation to anyone who'll take you. You wouldn't get a job that pays enough or develop your skills to increase your value in the marketplace since you feel doomed to failure. You wouldn't eat well because why bother if you think your unattractive anyway.

This type of thinking is an attack on your identity and destiny. Evil's agenda is simple: if she hates herself, then he can move on to someone else because self-hatred will breed much sin.

Love wants you to self-direct.

To self-direct is to shift the words inside to those words that can bring life.

> "We act in direct accordance with who we believe we are."

For more support, check out coach Robyn Coffman's helpful online program Beyond Skin Deep (*https://www.thecoffmancompany.online/beyondskindeep*).

Healing body shame is a major victory toward weight and eating freedom.

REFLECT & SHARE

1. How has a negative body image impacted your life?

   _____

   _____

2. What are some of the things that were said about your body that you need to heal?

   _____

   _____

3. Which Strategy most resonates for you?

   _____

   _____

4. How often do you judge and compare your body with others?

   _____

   _____

5. How can you better value who you are?

   _____

   _____

6. How does media influence how you feel about your body shape and size?

   _____

   _____

CHAPTER 20

KEYS TO WHOLE & FREE HEALTH

Some foods we run from like
we just saw an ex from high school.

We've taken every giant down. You've made it; enter your promised land! Remember weight and eating bondage to mold and shapes you to be Whole & Free..

Our job is to believe well and put action behind the Whole & Free us instead of the broken and bound version.

In this Chapter, I wanted to give you a few ways to make the transition a bit smoother from the old to the new for weight and eating freedom for life. Some points are reemphasized because they're important.

All in all, you have two books full of keys to clarify the meaning of Whole & Free Health. Each chapter seeks to elevate you mentally, spiritually, physically, and emotionally for your best life.

Persist until you win—until you are in the personal promised land you know is yours.

> " Our job is to believe well and put
> action behind the Whole & Free us instead
> of the broken and bound version. "

Your personal promised land is the biggest miracle of health transformation that you can see for yourself.

Keys to Whole & Free Health

The following guidelines are a mix of insights to embrace our wholeness and freedom. You no longer have to believe the lies about your body, yourself, or your food issues. Take heed to the keys as they will guide you to the full manifestation of the health that you're believing for.

Transition to the Life Abundant Standard

Nature created food for us to enjoy. Big Food created food for us to be enslaved. Nature created food for us to eat in abundance. Big Food created food for us to pay them an abundance in money. Think about it: to be enslaved to sugary soda or a crunchy chicken sandwich is all the evidence we need to know that we've been exploited.

We cannot truly enjoy food that has enslaved us.

> " **We cannot truly enjoy food that has enslaved us.** "

Foods that make us sick and tired have devastating consequences. They make us feel hopeless and powerless to change. In no way can these foods be claimed as loving.

This book is an order to win, not to dilly dally along. We're to come out of the Standard American Dietary ways that are killing us.

We cannot persist to obey our cravings for food that steal, kill, and destroy the body, mind, and spirit. The Standard American Diet is 84 percent processed, highly processed, and unclean foods based on both biblical and health principles, with only 16 percent fruits and vegetables. We're to increase our intake of real foods according to Genesis 1:29–30.

To transition out of this way of eating, we let go of false and fake foods and eat real and honest ones. S.A.D foods cause and create weight and eating bondage just as much as toxic shame does. It's important to reduce processed and fast food in our lives no matter our size or goals for the sole purpose of obedience and divine alignment.

We enjoy more of the abundant life when we align with God's

> It's important to reduce processed and fast food in our lives no matter our size or goals for the sole purpose of obedience and divine alignment.

abundant food.

Here are some reiterated ideas on how to transition from the S.A.D to the L.A.S.:

- Start right away or set a date to transition off a problem food or ingredient.
- Focus on what to eat, instead of what not to eat.
- Grow your amount of life abundant food intake over time.
- Find a new, non-media hobby to avoid food commercials and attacks on your body image that make us eat more.
- Replace problem foods with alternative versions.
- Increase the quality of your foods, especially your meats.
- Eat whole instead of refined grains.
- Focus on real foods.
- Prepare and eat more at home.
- Eliminate fast and processed foods.
- Never beat yourself up or condemn yourself for slip ups; they're to be expected.
- Keep learning.
- Don't expect to never overeat; stay away from extreme expectations with yourself.

- Take things one meal at a time.

- Set your intention by planning what to eat each day.

- Know that sometimes your inner glutton wins; keep going.

- Enjoy nurturing your body, soul, and spirit by applying Books 1 & 2.

Watch for All or Nothing Dieting Mindsets

A lifestyle change means daily efforts for the long haul. Diets are all or nothing—either on or off. All or nothing mindsets stem from unhealed trauma and a need to control. In Cognitive Behavioral Therapy (CBT) the all-or-nothing mindset is called a thinking distortion.

Do we need another diet? No.

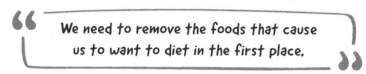

We need to remove the foods that cause us to want to diet in the first place.

We need to remove the foods that cause us to want to diet in the first place.

Earlier I said that the Standard American Diet is an eating disorder in itself. It's our addiction to this way of eating that causes us to want to diet (stop) eating it, but then we go back to it because it's addictive!

Therefore, our overarching goal to reduce and remove the foods is a lifestyle change that happens right now or over time if you need it to.

For freedom you'll need a defined food plan to be successful.

Explore food plans from Bright Line Eating, Food Addicts Anonymous, Chef AJ, Never Binge Again, or Mastering Diabetes to enhance your bio-individual food plan to have clear guidelines for what healthy eating looks like for you.

Pay attention to how you interact with problem foods. For example, if bread makes you revert to a full-fledged processed food lifestyle or you've had an on again off again relationship with it, try the whole grain option instead of the white refined option. Or eat two slices instead of the loaf. Or have bread once a week instead of daily.

If you find it to be nearly impossible to eat a portion once a week, then you know it's got to go. You'll be more successful in a healthy lifestyle if the ingredients of the bread are totally out of your system than you will doing an on again off again diet thing.

Diets are a distraction from true health transformation.

Most people swing from diet to diet or this tidbit of nutritional information to that tidbit only to get themselves all confused. Then they circle the mountain instead of casting it into the sea.

Watch out for the temptation to start new diets or fall into traps of this or that nutritional information like eat plums don't eat plums type of propaganda. Adhere to tried and true food truth to deter confusion and delay. Choose to adopt God's food truth in the Life Abundantly Standard for life.

Dieting behaviors are a sign of mental health problems as is untreated food addiction. Focus on daily health one meal at a time. Revisit Chapter 17 to Adopt the Freedom Mindset.

Heal Food Fear

When we're scared with anxieties around food, we have food fear. Some foods we run from like we just saw an ex from high school. If you feel like you can't trust yourself alone with a bag of cookies for example, you have food fear. In no way should any food make you feel afraid: "For God has not given us a spirit of fear, but of power and of love and of a sound mind" (2 Timothy 1:7).

Food fear shows up as:

- Fear of going out to eat
- Fear of being overwhelmed by your temptation to eat, overeat, or binge
- Fear of processed foods

- Fear of unhealthy foods
- Fear food groups (like carbs)

Take a moment to list out the foods that intimidate you—the ones that sit on the table and whisper your name in a creepy way. It's creepy because we know that cookies don't talk, so that voice comes from within.

Our fear of food is a sign of food addiction.

> **Our fear of food is a sign of food addiction.**

Food fear can be overcome through healing your inner glutton's needs, identifying the erroneous belief, addressing food addiction.

See, your inner glutton is really your inner child who doesn't believe she can hold up when faced with temptation, yet. She needs more healing to strengthen her resolve in who she is. Your healing words encourage her to know she doesn't have to go crazy and eat everything for fear that she won't be able to say no or stop. An Emotional Fitness Workout™ helps at the onset of food fear feelings.

Fear has an irrational belief under it too. An acronym is False Evidence Appearing Real (F.E.AR). Another one is Face Everything and Rise (F.E.A.R.). When you feel food fear, ask yourself, "What am I believing?" Then replace it with an affirmation that brings peace and causes you to raise your game.

Food addiction has a funny way of making us feel fearful of food or fearful of becoming out of control with it, especially during holidays and vacations. That's because we know it's our Pig. As Dr. Glenn Livingston would say, "We can cage the Pig!"

You have tools now. You don't have to be in fear about any food, nor do you need to harbor anger at the Standard American Diet.

Food fear can turn into another mental issue when we experience anxiety around foods. If you suspect you're overly health conscious, orthorexia nervosa is when health becomes rigid in your life.[1]

Orthorexia nervosa symptoms include:[2]

- Perfectionist, extremely rigid food control
- Inability to handle tricky food situations
- Undereating or restrictive eating
- Anxiety when faced with foods not considered healthy
- Self-imposed anxiety based on what they feel they can or can't eat

We want to get the problem foods out but not be overly rigid or filled with food fear.

For example, it's not never, ever eating a brownie again. It's not ever eating a brownie that's made from wheat and refined sugar because your addicted brain makes you eat more and more wheat and sugar.

It's also not being afraid of eating the brownie but choosing not to eat it due to your experience and history of eating brownies and their effects. Or you can decide to eat the brownie, enjoy it, and move on or to have less of it.

To get the S.A.D. out is good. Notice whether life revolves around being alone with our healthy foods, just as it can revolve around being alone with our unhealthy ones. We don't want to live for anything but the Lord.

Trust that you can make great food decisions even amid poor options.

Protect Your Environment

Food fear is one thing, but to protect your environment from temptation is wise. As Chef AJ says, "If it's in your house, it's in your mouth!"[3]

We do need to be mindful of tempting foods in our environment. We underestimate how protective it is to keep the binge foods and ingredients out of our homes.

If a food is tempting, get it out. Make it super inconvenient to attain it.

Your environment is powerful. See, when we're vulnerable from a long and tiresome workday, it's easy to ravish all the highly palatable food that's there.

> We underestimate how protective it is to keep
> the binge foods and ingredients out of our homes.

Humans can't help but choose the most densely energetic food in the environment.[4] We're wired to find the highest caloric food in the least amount of effort in the least amount of time.[5] Research proves that if given the option between a carrot and piece of celery, we'll choose the carrot. If given the option of a carrot or a piece of cake, we'll choose the cake.

I don't know a clearer explanation for wasted produce.

Keep the junk out so that you choose optimally. For more insights on living with a food addict, check out my blog on *www.thechubby-church.com*.

How can you better protect your environment from foods that don't support your wellbeing?

Be Patient

Many desire to be healed and whole this instant. They do one or two therapy sessions and kick themselves for not being how they think they should be. I've seen dozens of people get frustrated with themselves and God because they're not healed yet.

God is perfecting us and will finish the work in us until He comes (Philippians 1:6).

There is no end date on healing. It's a lifelong process.

There are only levels or phases of healing. And to be frustrated because you need more healing in an area you thought you solved is soul shame. Soul shame always lets us know we're not good enough—that we should be done with the granola bar binges already.

If you've been in weight and eating bondage for years, give healing some time. It takes time because to come out of weight and eating bondage is also to come out of bondage—period.

Be patient with yourself as you learn your needs. As the soul heals, our eating habits adjust and weight stabilizes. You love your body and soul right out of shame.

If you feel the need to rush to lose weight, you've fallen into a dieter's mindset. So, don't make attempts to drop ten pounds in a week. Instead put in place actions that support change. There is no end date on healthy living. As you make healthful daily choices, you'll manifest your healthiest body, soul, and spirit.

> " *To come out of weight and eating bondage is also to come out of bondage—period.* "

Celebrate All Along the Way

Celebrate the progress you're making and have made all along the way. When soul shame tempts you to beat yourself up over the mistake you made, your Whole & Free you is cheering you on for all of your efforts, big and small.

Celebrate:

- Your binges shrunk in calorie load (You've gone from 2,000 calories to 250 calories.)
- You no longer wallow in self-pity or beat yourself up for mistakes.
- If you do wallow in self-pity and beat yourself up, you don't do so as long.
- You don't manifest your inner glutton at the same frequency.
- You no longer diet or get duped by get-skinny-quick ads.
- You're on track more often.
- You no longer use food to cope and don't emotionally eat over things you used to.
- You identify your addictive voice and more times than not you don't listen to it.
- Every time you don't listen to your addicted voice.
- You went from a binge daily to bi-weekly.

- Your sugar demon is quiet.
- You wear clothes that fit.
- You've upgraded your food quality.
- You downsized from the family-sized portion to a personal-sized one.

Bust out your theme song and dance. You're changing! I'd love to hear that you're celebrating all your successes in every area of life. Increase the amount of celebration for your life, and you'll have a life to celebrate!

Focus on Health Not Weight

Keep your focus on health. *Be* healthy. When you believe you're healthy, you do healthy actions and manifest healthy results.

> " Increase the amount of celebration for your life, and you'll have a life to celebrate! "

What we give words to we give life to. We don't want to be controlled by our weight, so we need to reduce its influence in our lives and give it less of our thought life attention as a problem. Think about what you think about. If health, weight, or food takes up most of your thought life, it will pose to be most of our life's problems. As you reduce your thoughts on weight and food and instead do actions to meal plan and take great care of yourself, weight and food will become less of a problem.

What we focus on expands.

You can reduce your focus on weight by not saying things like, "Oh, I'm so fat," or, "I need to lose weight." Talk about all you're doing to live into your identity in health. Keep your healthy actions focused on health, not weight loss efforts.

On the flipside, if weight discussions have been a taboo part of soul shame, be bold and share more about what's really happening for you in your weight.

Weight fluctuates up and down all day long. It's a very complicated metric and can limit us psychologically if we get stuck on it. To measure changes, use measures that make sense, such as body fat, before and after photos each month of progress, waist or hip measurements, or clothing size.

Keep your focus on doing healthy actions, believing that you are a healthy person and being healthy.

Make Time To Sit and Eat

You've been there, driving with your knee, managing to get a bite of that delicious bacon cheeseburger while manually shifting gears with fallen crumbs in the crevasses that even the best car detailers can't seem to get to. Or is that just me?

You know my Burger King story, but McDonalds, Wendy's, and Chick-fil-A have hung out in my car too. The car should be *the car*, not the table, restaurant, or picnic, but for many of us it's our dining space.

The National Highway Traffic Safety Administration reported 80 percent of accidents and 65 percent of near misses are caused by foods, with burgers and coffee being involved most often.[6]

We make time to eat when we eat less in the car, bus, or—if you're really a rebel—the motorcycle. Imagine that.

Certainly store (non-binge inducing) healthy options in the glove compartment so that you don't get over hungry when having a long drive or one of those hectic days. Better on-hand options prevent ravished eating later.

But yes, you can make time to eat mindfully by eating more at home. I realize at home could mean in your bed, on the couch, or in your home office. But do consider eating at the table.

Take a moment to sit down and eat.

When we eat at the table, it's an act of nurturance. When you eat, do it consciously and slowly. Sit your bum in a chair and savor the flavors.

Furthermore, dining with others helps us to be more mindful to sit and eat. It also helps us to focus on connecting with people more than food. Eat a few meals with the family each week or invite friends over to sit at the table and enjoy the fellowship.

Help Others

When we help others in an area we struggle with, we'll see the struggle end. Helping others who struggle promotes our best health because we feel accountable.

Help by sharing this content with others. Be the wellness advocate in your family. Host a book club to process through the Reflect & Share questions together. Share a chapter with someone else.

We don't start to help after we implement everything. We start to help now so that everything is easier to implement. As we help others, we heal ourselves. So why not start today? How can you help others to get Whole & Free?

> As we help others, we heal ourselves.

Pride Puffs Up

Have you ever said, "I've been good today," in regard to how you've eaten?

The shame and pride in us make us think that we're good or bad depending on how we eat. And you're not good or bad based on how you eat or what you eat.

You're good, period. But we can be arrogant or humble in our pursuits in health.

Either are a sign of being broken and bound, not Whole & Free. Spirit is stabilizing your identity through your health journey. And one of the best pieces of advice I can offer is to watch out for pride that puffs up. In other words, stay humble.

Oftentimes we get in our best bodies and act the fool. Have you been there before?

We reveal lots of skin, think we're better than others, or have this *I've arrived* mindset, so we start eating like we used to and

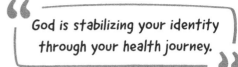

God is stabilizing your identity through your health journey.

come back to the same base of the mountain we were at when we started. We're healing our identity. We need to get the arrogance out so that our worth and value isn't based on how we look or what size we wear.

Many wear chubby suits because of the shame of the trauma, along with body and soul shame, but also because of the shamelessness of our eating.

We don't humble our mouths.

Shamelessness is pride and arrogance. Shame and shamelessness (pride) operate together. They both come from a soul of worthlessness, which gathers worth from things outside of God's love. Don't wait to feel worthy or valuable to eat right. Our worth isn't in our size or how we eat; it's found in love alone.

Some ways arrogance and pride show up in our weight and eating matters are:

- In denial about the severity of food addiction in our lives

Shame and shamelessness (pride) operate together.

- Continuing to engage in foods you know are an idol
- Too much time in the gym, with mirrors, or social media selfies
- Not satisfied with our bodies how they are
- Obsessed with attaining a smaller and smaller size after achieving healthy weight
- Focus moves from healthy to "skinny" focus
- Over attention to clothing, make up, and looks
- Immodesty, wearing revealing clothing
- Superiority demonstrated by comments or judgments about others viewed as less than

- Judging what others eat
- Conceited comments about looks and body
- Showing off your body
- Not giving any effort because we think we've arrived

Any of these items are a manifestation of a soul that needs to heal. When you sense any of them, it's a call to heal. We heal pride by humbling ourselves and doing the soul healing work.

To get comfortable in our right-sized bodies is also to get comfortable in a humble soul. Let us make sure that we don't have any food idols or pride there.

Embrace the Whole & Free You

It's a bit weird to go through life without the drama of weight and eating struggles at first. You don't have to get your love and comfort from supremely succulent snacks or rush to the gym to work it off for several hours. It's sweet to just have a drama free, less exciting life in that way.

You get to create your life and its outcomes.

Who are you now that you don't have a weight and eating problem? Who are you now that you can hear your soul speak amongst the beast, the lies, and the emotions?

Who do you want to be?

What do you want to build?

As you move out of the weight and eating struggle, you embrace the Whole & Free you. Review recommendations, and put them in place one at a time until successful.

You've been Whole & Free this whole time. Only the lies—have infiltrated your truth with this smokescreen of a broken and bound identity that you've lived in. You don't have to choose foods that don't serve your highest good. You don't have to eat to fit in at gatherings. You can stand in your truth. You can stand food truth.

As Dr Seuss said, "Why fit in when you were born to stand out?"[7]

And as Jesus said, "Let your light so shine before men, that they may see your good works and glorify your Father in heaven" (Matthew 5:16).

You're Whole & Free When

- You believe that you're Whole & Free.
- You have nothing to hide, including your soul.
- You have dealt what you need to from the past.
- Your actions, thoughts, and words are aligned and congruent.
- You don't engage with behaviors that bring shame, guilt, and regret.
- You have faith in God and yourself to come through on your word and desires.
- You no longer have an out of control, high control nature, but there's an excellence and rest that you do things out of, not out of a place of striving.
- Your worth is not in how much you weigh, how you look, or any other performance metric but in love.
- You don't fear man, food, or rejection.
- You can manage your life (financials, household, responsibilities, and possessions).
- You help others to become Whole & Free.

Do the Work

Don't we deserve what we work for? Our truest desires are backed up with actions. And life rewards those actions. People who work toward health will be blessed with better health.

We sow and we reap.

If we sow the wrong way into our bodies, we'll continue to reap depression, emotional instability, body shame, and fatigue. Every time

> If we sow the wrong way into our bodies, we'll continue to reap depression, emotional instability, body shame, and fatigue.

we choose the sweet-deceiving enemy's table and we sow the wrong seeds. If we don't change our choices, we'll harvest aches and pains.

We're double minded when we say that we want to be free but treat our body poorly.

When actions align with words, we get results. Faith without works is dead. Faith in health is demonstrated by healthy choices and actions— by sowing well.

Our bodies are the number one thing we sow into. More valuable than money, our bodies are what we steward the most.

Take the parable of the talents: the one rewarded was the one who made the most of the investment given. He took the ten denarii and multiplied it.

He invested. He sowed. He trusted.

All of this is action.

For the right actions he was rewarded with more.

Action creates outcomes.

We can't play victim and be like the sower who didn't advance the investment.

It would feel like a waste to give the organic dish to the person who doesn't care if they eat organic or not. Why would I waste time and energy giving super thoughtful, health-conscious meals to people who could care less about how they treat their bodies?

We give to those who make effort, who sow, and who do what they're supposed to do.

To sow poorly is a disguise for obeying temptation.

The remedy to end excuses is to choose not to have any excuses. No more playing victim to temptation. You are victorious. Bless your body. Bless your soul. Bless your spirit.

Next up is to read ***The Chubby Church Book 2: An Order to Win the 7 Battles of the Weight & Eating War for Good!*** To go your next level in freedom you'll need to address giants of

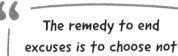

> **The remedy to end excuses is to choose not to have any excuses.**

food addiction, overeating, unclean eating, and more. You can order it now on amazon, audible, or kindle. Or go to www.thechubbychurch.com. Thank you so much for reading and reviewing. Thank you for your grace with my deep devotion to Christ as a Christ-centered minister.

You are Whole & Free, walk in it.

REFLECT & SHARE

1. Which Whole & Free Health keys spoke to you the most?

_____

_____

_____

2. What can you do to protect yourself from eating mishaps?

_____

_____

_____

3. How has arrogance affected you in the past?

_____

_____

_____

INVITATION TO CHRIST

Churches are like restaurants: you've got to try them until you find a favorite.

Have you ever had a house guest ruin your home's atmosphere? Maybe he or she criticized every little thing or brought nasty music, nasty food, nasty ways, and a nasty attitude into your dwelling space? This is how I liken a holy God—our God, who is love.

Certain people just can't understand, receive, or interpret the presence of God. Like that house guest, who couldn't get your loving atmosphere, needed to go, so also the cancers of hate, negativity, pride, and other stinky attitudes would need to depart from an atmosphere of holiness, peace, and love.

God sent Jesus for us to be able to reconcile with God through Jesus because the Father is too holy for us to bear. He is so holy that we would die in His presence unless He sent us a redeeming branch to cover our unholiness and ridiculousness so that we can be reconciled to the Holy One. Jesus is our olive branch.

We get to be adopted to a heavenly, holy Father, through His Son, by the power of the Holy Spirit.

One thing is for sure: "For God so loved the world that He gave His only begotten Son, that whoever believes in Him should not perish but have everlasting life" (John 3:16). God absolutely loves you and is excited about you! He wants you on His team. He wants to help you with this thing called life. He wants to teach you how to love, grow, and help yourself, your family, and others.

He gives the free gift of salvation, which is an invitation to His kingdom. He's already Lord, but we just want to acknowledge Him in our lives and come into alignment with the true Lover of our souls.

Douglas Groothuis, researcher and author of *Christian Apologetics* said, "He [Jesus] entered the world supernaturally, accredited Himself with unparalleled signs and wonders, possessed an impeccable character, made claims only befitting God Himself, and died with the purpose of redeeming humanity. The best account of the historical facts is that He was who He said He was. If this is so, we should respond to Him on His terms[1]... Other gods are prophets, not messiahs, avatars, not incarnate, sages, not saviors."[2]

And because God is so good, all you need to do is bring your words and heart into alignment by confession, then seek out a church to get baptized as soon as possible for the remission of sins in the name of Jesus Christ—who signs the check on our salvation.

Baptism is a sign that you've now entered the kingdom of God and are partnering with the Holy Spirit to bring about your true identity and purpose in the earth.

Will you pray the prayer on the next page to acknowledge the Lord? As Romans 10:8-11 instructs, "If you confess with your mouth the Lord Jesus and believe in your heart that God has raised Him from the dead, you will be saved. For with the heart one believes unto righteousness, and with the mouth confession is made unto salvation. For the Scripture says, 'Whoever believes in Him will not be put to shame'".

DAYSTAR NETWORK'S PRAYER FOR SALVATION[3]

"Dear Lord Jesus,

I know that according to your Word in John 3:3, I must be born again to see the kingdom of God. Father I know I am a sinner. I believe Christ died for me. I believe that you shed your blood, died on the cross for me, and rose again from the dead. I repent and turn from my sins. I need you, Jesus.

I no longer want to be in control of my life. Please come into my heart, forgive me of my sins, and be my personal Lord and Savior from this day forward. Please give me the strength by your precious Holy Spirit to live for you.

Please forgive me of my sins … I want to turn from my sins.

Jesus, thank you for the gift of salvation. I promise to obey you with the help of the Holy Spirit and to follow you all the days of my life. In Jesus's name, amen."

For resources for your confession go to:

https://howtoknowjesus.joycemeyer.org/
http://www.daystar.com/prayer/know-jesus/

Check out various churches in your local area until you find one that feels right for you. Churches are like restaurants: you've got to try them until you find a favorite. Get a good Bible that you can understand and enjoy your new adventure with the Lord!

Congratulations! Your life will never be the same again.

Welcome to the team! If you've prayed this prayer, please email:

info@wholeandfreepress.com.

ACKNOWLEDGEMENTS

I am deeply thankful to the many people that have prayed over this work, contributed to this work, supported me in the work, and who received the work. I could not have done this without your prayers, love, encouragement, kindness, beta reading, proof-reading, editing, teaching, training, patience, coaching, and generosity that saw me through. I'll trust you know who you are. Few days go by that I don't thank God for laying me on your heart for prayer or support to see His plan through.

I love you.

Thank you! Thank you! Thank you!

NON-EDIBLE GOODIES

SEAS - Self-Esteem Inventory

DIRECTIONS: For each of the statements below, rate what is your level of exhibiting these behaviors in your life. Use the following rating scale and circle the number of your rating for each item:

1 = never   2 = rarely   3 = sometimes   4 = frequently   5 = almost always

1. I seek approval and affirmation from others, and I am afraid of criticism.

    1   2   3   4   5

2. I guess at what normal behavior is, and I usually feel as if I am different from other people.

    1   2   3   4   5

3. I isolate myself from and am afraid of people in authority roles.

    1   2   3   4   5

4. I am not able to appreciate my own accomplishments and good deeds.

    1   2   3   4   5

5. I tend to have difficulty following a project through from beginning to end.

    1   2   3   4   5

6. I get frightened or stressed when I am in the company of an angry person.

    1   2   3   4   5

7. In order to avoid a conflict, I find it easier to lie than tell the truth.

    1   2   3   4   5

8. I have problems with my own compulsive behavior, e.g., drinking, drug use, gambling, overeating, smoking, use of sex, shopping, etc.

1   2   3   4   5

9. I judge myself without mercy. I am my own worst critic, and I am harder on myself than I am on others.

1   2   3   4   5

10. I feel more alive in the midst of a crisis, and I am uneasy when my life is going smoothly; I am continually anticipating problems.

1   2   3   4   5

11. I have difficulty having fun. I don't seem to know how to play for fun and relaxation.

1   2   3   4   5

12. I am attracted to others whom I perceive to have been victims, and I develop close relationships with them. In this way I confuse love with pity, and I love people I can pity and rescue.

1   2   3   4   5

13. I need perfection in my life at home and work, and I expect perfection from others in my life.

1   2   3   4   5

14. I seek out novelty, excitement, and the challenge of newness in my life with little concern given to the consequences of such action.

1   2   3   4   5

15. I take myself very seriously, and I view all of my relationships just as seriously.

1   2   3   4   5

16. I have problems developing and maintaining intimate relationships.

1   2   3   4   5

17. I feel guilty when I stand up for myself or take care of my needs first, instead of giving in or taking care of others' needs first.

               1   2   3   4   5

18. I seek and/or attract people who have compulsive behaviors (e.g., alcohol, drugs, gambling, food, shopping, sex, smoking, overworking, or seeking excitement.)

               1   2   3   4   5

19. I feel responsible for others and find it easier to have concern for others than for myself.

               1   2   3   4   5

20. I am loyal to people for whom I care, even in the face of evidence that the loyalty is undeserved.

               1   2   3   4   5

21. I cling to and will do anything to hold on to relationships because I am afraid of being alone and fearful of being abandoned.

               1   2   3   4   5

22. I am impulsive and act too quickly, before considering alternative actions or possible consequences.

               1   2   3   4   5

23. I have difficulty in being able to feel or to express feelings; I feel out of touch with my feelings.

               1   2   3   4   5

24. I mistrust my feelings and the feelings expressed by others.

               1   2   3   4   5

25. I isolate myself from other people, and I am initially shy and withdrawn in new social settings.

               1   2   3   4   5

26. I feel that I am being taken advantage of by individuals and society in general; I often feel victimized.

$$1 \quad 2 \quad 3 \quad 4 \quad 5$$

27. I can be overresponsible much of the time, but I can be extremely irresponsible at other times.

$$1 \quad 2 \quad 3 \quad 4 \quad 5$$

28. I feel confused and angry at myself and not in control of my environment or my life when the stresses are great.

$$1 \quad 2 \quad 3 \quad 4 \quad 5$$

29. I spend a lot of time and energy rectifying or cleaning up my messes and the negative consequences of ill-thought-out or impulsive actions for which I am responsible.

$$1 \quad 2 \quad 3 \quad 4 \quad 5$$

30. I deny that my current problems stem from my past life. I deny that I have stuffed-in feelings from the past which are impeding my current life.

$$1 \quad 2 \quad 3 \quad 4 \quad 5$$

Scoring and Interpretation

Add the ratings for all 30 items in your journal. This score indicates the degree to which you are affected by low self-esteem.

Score Interpretation

0-30 | Not affected by low self-esteem.

31-45 | Traces of low self-esteem. Take preventive action to reduce its impact on your life.

46-61 | Presence of mild low self-esteem in your life. Take steps to treat this.

62-90 | Presence of moderate low self-esteem. Take steps to treat this as soon as possible.

91-120 | Presence of severe low self-esteem. Take steps to treat this immediately.

121-150 | Presence of profound low self-esteem. Take immediate step to treat this and seek out professional help to assist you in this process.

http://coping.us/seasmanual/selfesteeminventory.html

A Prayer of Gratitude for the Body

- Lord thank you for my toes and feet. Thank you for giving me feet that take me in the direction you send me. Thank you that I have feet to stand on. Thank you that my feet are blessed and shod with the gospel of peace.

- Lord thank you for my legs. Lord I could not have any legs to stand on. Thank you for giving me legs to help get me where you want me to go. Thank you for my knees that help me to sit and bend. Thank you for my thighs, help me to accept them as they are, and see them as the strength that they are for my body.

- Lord thank you for my hips. Thank you that I am able to sit comfortably. Thank you that I get to have this body and the ability to move and choose clothing that helps me to feel confident.

- Thank you Lord for your protection over my body and over my shape and size as it is. Thank you that you accept me for the body I have. Lord help me to accept this body you gave me. Help me to love what you have created in me and in this body. Thank you, Father, for anointing me with the grace and strength to honor my body.

- Lord I repent for harm and abuse to my body and I ask you to help me to treat it as a Holy Vessel of your spirit. I ask you to help me to appreciate it and to value it. Thank you, Lord, for this temporary home of my body that helps me to implement your will on earth.

- Thank you Father for my stomach. Thank you that I have digestion and organs that are working. Thank you for the stomach I have, it could be bigger, it could be flatter, but it's functioning and its mine. Please nourish me from your spirit and help me to love my stomach. I ask you to help me accept my stomach exactly how it is.

- Thank you, Father, for freeing me from criticism of my body! Thank you for helping me to stop negatively evaluating my body shape and size. Thank you for helping me not to dwell on worldly things.

- Thank you, Father, for my arms. Thank you that they help me to pick things up, hug those I love, carry my bags, and put myself in more comfortable conditions. Thank you for the arms that give me strength. Thank you for my hands Father! Thank you for my fingers and my nails. Thank you that I can work with these hands, I can feel with these hands, I can Facebook with these typing fingers. I can cook and eat with these hands. I can praise your name with these hands! I can lift my hands up to you.

- Thank you for my neck that turns my head.

- Thank you for the weight I have on my body. Thank you that I am not being carried out of my house due to obesity. Thank you for increasing my appreciation for my current body size and shape exactly how it is. Thank you, Father, for setting me free from weight and eating bondage. Thank you for setting me free from valuing myself based on my weight! Thank you for freedom from being weight obsessive. Thank you that my body can hold weight. Thank you that my body can release weight.

- Thank you that the head is the authority over the body. Thank you for my brain that communicates to my body and organs what to do and when to it. Thank you, Father, for my face. Thank you for my eyes, eyebrows, lips, and nose. Thank you for the senses I get to experience that involve my head. Thank you for my head's shape and size. Thank you for the value of my brain, that I can do things, and help others with it.

- Thank you, Body, for all of your remarkable service to my soul and spirit. Thank you, my Body, for forgiveness for the damage I've done to you. You are alive! I will treat you with love and care!

- Thank God for those parts of the body that you struggle to fully appreciate, value, and accept. Thank God for the hair on your head, or the hair you may have left, or your head shaped for baldness. Thank God even for your private parts. Thank God for your organs, your heart, liver, and kidneys for example. Thank God even for those unique birthmarks, beauty marks, and scars. Turn around your body hatred to body appreciation.

Emotional Fitness Workout™ Worksheet

Use this worksheet to move through the steps in Chapter 18.

1	Stop

2	Pinpoint

3	Evaluate

4	Experience

5	Release

Emotional Fitness Workout™ Worksheet

Use this worksheet to move through the steps in Chapter 18.

1	Stop

2	Pinpoint

3	Evaluate

4	Experience

5	Release

What is the Standard American Diet?[3]

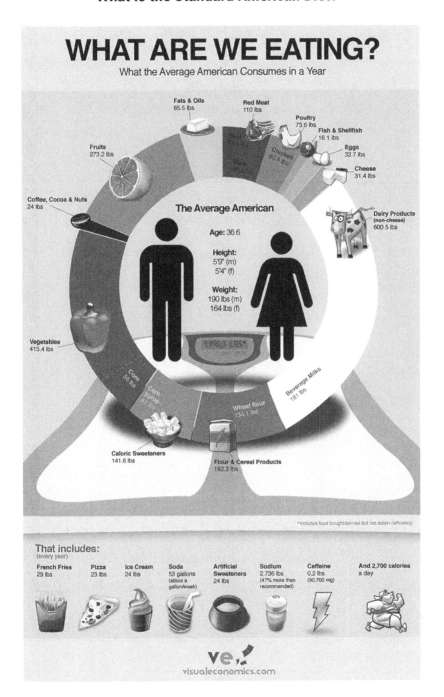

WHAT ARE WE EATING?

What the Average American Consumes in a Year

Fats & Oils
85.5 lbs

Red Meat
110 lbs

Poultry
73.6 lbs

Fish & Shellfish
16.1 lbs

Eggs
32.7 lbs

Cheese
31.4 lbs

Fruits
273.2 lbs

Coffee, Cocoa & Nuts
24 lbs

The Average American

Age: 36.6

Height:
5'9" (m)
5'4" (f)

Weight:
190 lbs (m)
164 lbs (f)

Dairy Products
(non-cheese)
600.5 lbs

Vegetables
415.4 lbs

1,996.3 LBS*

Corn
56 lbs

Corn Syrup
42 lbs

Wheat flour
134.1 lbs

Beverage Milks
181 lbs

Caloric Sweeteners
141.6 lbs

Flour & Cereal Products
192.3 lbs

*Includes food bought/served but not eaten (leftovers)

That includes:
(every year)

| French Fries | Pizza | Ice Cream | Soda | Artificial Sweeteners | Sodium | Caffeine | And 2,700 calories |
| 29 lbs | 23 lbs | 24 lbs | 53 gallons (about a gallon/week) | 24 lbs | 2,736 lbs (47% more than recommended) | 0.2 lbs (90,700 mg) | a day |

ve
visualeconomics.com

329

Body Honor Manifesto

Whole & Free Health
Regarding my body, I…

Talk kindly
"I only talk kindly to my body."

Thank it
"I'm thankful for my body."

Accept it
"I accept my body as it is."

Enjoy i
"I enjoy life in my body."

Trust it
"I trust my body."

Listen to it
"I listen to my body."

Heal it
"I heal my body."

Look at it
"I look at myself with eyes of appreciation."

Love it
"My body is scared and special. I love it."

UPCOMING BOOKS

Follow me on Amazon to be notified of upcoming books!

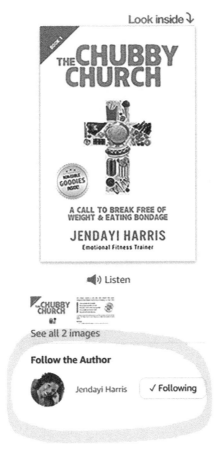

Look up The Chubby Church then click "Follow the Author"
or click the following link:
https://www.amazon.com/Jendayi-Harris/e/
B07Q5NMWQM?ref_=dbs_p_pbk_r00_abau_000000

Are you in need of hope for a close relationship?

After over 20 years of relational conflict between mother and daughter, God did a miracle healing in the life of Jendayi's mother, Joann.

Undiagnosed is a beautiful story of a redeemed mother and daughter relationship in Christ Jesus. In this memoir, Jendayi shares the process of healing and how God answers prayer, heals addiction, and restores family.

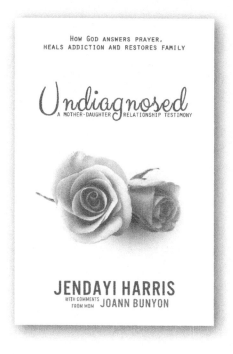

HOW GOD ANSWERS PRAYER,
HEALS ADDICTION AND RESTORES FAMILY

Undiagnosed
A MOTHER-DAUGHTER & RELATIONSHIP TESTIMONY

JENDAYI HARRIS
WITH COMMENTS FROM MOM JOANN BUNYON

How is your Self-Talk?

- Are you tired of struggling with not doing what you know better to do?
- Do you talk yourself into poor choices that you regret later?
- Do you feel you need to obey the voice in your head?
- The missing foundational link to creating true freedom and wholeness – practically

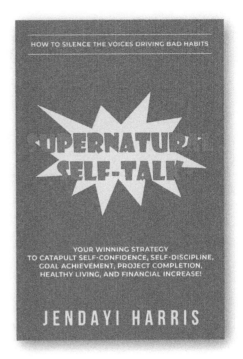

In this short read, Supernatural Self-Talk, Jendayi uses Biblical principles, stories, and practical tips, this book will help build your self-talk to support your best well-being and to develop more supportive, connected conversations within yourself and with others. If you beat yourself, have trouble letting go of things you don't want to do, or have the need for inner healing get this book! It will change your inner world which will manifest in your outer world.

Follow Jendayi Harris on Amazon to be notified of new books.

For Moms Who:

- Have regrets from early experiences raising their children
- Feel hurt or distant from her adult child
- Need strategies to stop beating herself up with guilt
- Want to improve her relationship with herself and her adult child

Are you a mom with regrets from early experiences as mothers, and who feel the consequences in their current relationships with their adult child?

This book is a big hug for you! In this book, I talk about an 8-step strategy your adult child needs to repair your relationship.

Instead of beating yourself up with guilt, feeling angry that your adult child is disconnected from you, or worrying about seeing your grandchildren – Take Action! The book and workbook together pack a powerful strategy to take back your family!

Follow Jendayi on Amazon to hear of new releases.

Are You Emotionally Fit?

You'll learn:

- How to understand emotions and get ego out of the way
- The 5-step Emotional Fitness Workout™ for inner strength to feel happy, healthy, and whole for life
- Why so many religious people fail to show the love of God
- How to navigate the triggers that sabotage relationships

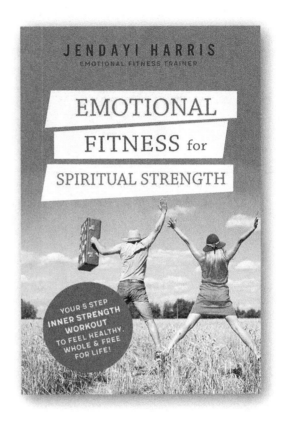

Spiritual and religious communities know that something is missing when a person isn't willing to work on their character, reactions, and general personal development.

Using Biblical principles, stories, and practical tips, this book will help build your emotional body to ward off offense, fear, and anger, and to develop more connected conversations and a loving presence.

Follow Jendayi on Amazon to hear of new releases.

Too busy to read?
Listen to Book 2 instead on:

an **amazon** company

www.audible.com

Did you enjoy *Whole & Free Health*?

I need your help to get the word out!

Will you help?

Your review helps others decide to purchase this book on *www.Amazon.com*.

Thank you!

Post your review today!

Join Whole & Free Health to

- Share in *The Chubby Church* reading experience
- Have a place to share your successes
- Find products that work for others for cleansing and supplementation
- Share recipes
- Share and receive devotionals, prayers, and encouragement
- Get accountability
- Meet others who share the journey
- Join optional paid courses – Whole & Free Health Body, Whole & Free Health Soul, or Whole & Free Health Spirit. You can choose online and live workshops as available, to focus on applying *The Chubby Church* book contents and more
- Join optional paid audio-visual book club for Jendayi to read to you

It's FREE!

Go to: *www.Facebook.com*
Search: Whole and Free Health

Jendayi Harris is a minister of practical advice on how to do life in Christ well. She has a Bachelor of Science in Business Administration from Seton Hall University as a part of the distinguished Martin Luther King Scholarship Association. She received her Master of Arts in Counseling Psychology from Colorado Christian University. She's a Nationally Certified Counselor, as well as a Licensed Professional Counselor in Colorado. After a health revelation in her early twenties, she became a Board-Certified Health Coach with the Institute of Integrative Nutrition.

From a Ministry standpoint, she has been mentored by Rabbi Ralph Messer of Simchat Torah Beit Midrash, Pastor Tayo Obigbesan of Christ Liberty Restoration Ministries and is now an active member of BridgeWay Church under Pastor Peter Young and Apostle Bill Johnson of Bethel Church.

Jendayi is certified as a DiSc instructor with TTI and a Certified Emotional Intelligence facilitator from industry leader, Talent Smart. In her leisure time she enjoys teaching, writing, family, running, and her husband, gospel artist and music director Dr. Michael A. Williams, Sr.

Her unique background and experience in many areas as well as incredible life experience makes her a source of Godly practical advice and wisdom in an age of information and great confusion.

As a Soul Freedom Author & Teacher, she speaks on a range of topics and issues of soul and family restoration. In her opinion, to love God, your self, and others, is the most productive response to our daily insanity.

To hire her for speaking or to hear about her latest releases, visit her site at

www.jendayiharris.com.

Photograph by Kymora Jaxson Photography

NOTES

Introduction

1. Stephanie Averkamp, "Diet and Weight Loss Statistics,"
    fitnessforweightloss.com, accessed March 16, 2019, *http://www.*
    fitnessforweightloss.com/diet-and-weight-loss-statistics/.

Chapter 2: Gaining Whole & Free Health

1. Eric A. Finkelstein et al., "Obesity and Severe Obesity Forecasts through
    2030," American Journal of Preventive Medicine 42 (6) (2012): 563–
    70, *https://doi.org/10.1016/j.amepre.2011.10.026.*

2. Alexandros N. Vgontzas et al., "Obesity and Self-Reported Short Sleep
    Duration: A Marker of Sleep Complaints and Chronic Psychosocial
    Stress," Sleep Medicine Clinics 4, no. 1 (2009): 65–75, accessed April
    24, 2018. doi:10.1016/j.jsmc.2009.01.001.

3. "Adult Obesity Facts | Overweight & Obesity | CDC," Centers for
    Disease Control and Prevention, accessed March 16, 2019, *https://www.*
    cdc.gov/obesity/data/adult.html.

4. Claire Y. Wang et al., "Health and Economic Burden of the Projected
    Obesity Trends in the USA and the UK," The Lancet 378, no. 9793
    (August 27, 2011): 815–825, doi:10.1016/s0140-6736(11)60814-3.

5. Jessica Glenza, 2017, "Only One in 10 Americans Eat
    Enough Fruits and Vegetables, CDC Study Finds," The
    Guardian, Guardian News and Media, November 17,
    2017, https://www.theguardian.com/us-news/2017/nov/17/
    just-12-of-americans-eat-enough-fruit-and-vegetables-cdc-study-finds.

6. Federation of American Societies for Experimental Biology (FASEB),
    "Highly Processed Foods Dominate U.S. Grocery Purchases,"
    Science Daily, March 29, 2015, *http://www.sciencedaily.com/*
    releases/2015/03/150329141017.htm.

7. "Denial," Merriam-Webster, accessed March 17, 2019, *https://www.merriam*-webster.com/dictionary/denial.

Chapter 3: Welcome to Burger King – My Story

1. Kevin Trudeau, *Natural Cures They Don't Want You to Know About* (Elks Grove Village, IL: Alliance Publishing Group, 2004).

Chapter 4: Do You Want Freedom with That?

1. Watchman Nee, *The Spiritual Man* (Anaheim, CA: Living Stream Ministry, 1998).

2. Sanctify." n.d. Merriam-Webster accessed April 28, 2019. *https://www.merriam-webster.com/dictionary/sanctify.*

3. Nicholas Bakalar, "37.2 Trillion: Galaxies or Human Cells?" *The New York Times,* December 21, 2017, *https://www.nytimes.com/2015/06/23/science/37-2-trillion-galaxies-or-human-cells.html.*

4. Watchman Nee, *The Spiritual Man*, 198.

5. American Psychiatric Association, *Diagnostic and Statistical Manual of Mental Disorders: DSM-5.* 5th ed. (Arlington, VA: American Psychiatric Association, 2013).

6. Henry Wright, *A More Excellent Way* (New Kensington, PA: Whitaker House, 2009).

Chapter 5: The Call to Weight & Eating Freedom Action Plan

1. Stephanie Averkamp, "Diet and Weight Loss Statistics," fitnessforweightloss.com, accessed March 16, 2019, *http://www.fitnessforweightloss.com/diet-and-weight-loss-statistics/.*

2. Lysa TerKeurst, Made to Crave: Satisfying Your Deepest Desire with God, Not Food: Six Sessions: Participants Guide (Grand Rapids, MI: Zondervan, 2011), 11.

3. Amy Osmond Cook, "Healthy Living: Defeating the Couch Potato," Orange County Register, October 23, 2014, *https://www.ocregister.com/2014/10/23/healthy-living-defeating-the-couch-potato/.*

4. Ibid.

5. William Arthur Ward, "If You Can Imagine It, You Can Achieve It. If You Can Dream It, You Can Become It," accessed March 17, 2019, *https://www.quotes.net/quote/6643.*

6. *Alcoholics Anonymous* (New York: Works Pub., 1948).

7. Ibid.

8. Swimcoachpro, "Increase Your Chances of Achieving Your GOALs by up to 95%," Swimcoach, October 17, 2018, *https://swimcoach-pro.com/2018/04/30/increase-your-chances-of-achieving-your-goals-by-up-to-95/.*

Chapter 6: Master Body Care

1. National Center for Chronic Disease Prevention and Health Promotion (NCCDPHP), "Health and Economic Costs of Chronic Diseases," Centers for Disease Control and Prevention, February 11, 2019, accessed February 27, 2019, *https://www.cdc.gov/chronicdisease/about/costs/index.htm.*

2. Ibid.

3. CDC Newsroom, "Up to 40 Percent of Annual Deaths from Each of Five Leading U.S. Causes Are Preventable," Centers for Disease Control and Prevention, May 1, 2014, accessed February 27, 2019, *https://www.cdc.gov/media/releases/2014/p0501-preventable-deaths.html.*

4. "Introduction," Dietary Guidelines 2015–2020, accessed February 27, 2019, *https://health.gov/dietaryguidelines/2015/guidelines/introduction/nutrition-and-health-are-closely-related/.*

5. Pam Belluck, "Children's Life Expectancy Being Cut Short by Obesity," *The New York Times,* March 17, 2005, accessed March 25, 2017, *https://www.nytimes.com/2005/03/17/health/childrens-life-expectancy-being-cut-short-by-obesity.html.*

6. "Mental Illness," National Institute of Mental Health, November 2017, accessed February 27, 2019, *https://www.nimh.nih.gov/health/statistics/mental-illness.shtml.*

7. "50% of Mentally Ill Untreated," Mental Illness Policy Org, accessed February 27, 2019, *https://mentalillnesspolicy.org/consequences/percentage-mentally-ill-untreated.html*

8. Rosalynn Carter, Rebecca Palpant Shimkets, and Thomas H. Bornemann, "Creating and Changing Public Policy to Reduce the Stigma of Mental Illness," *Psychological Science in the Public Interest* 15, No. 2 (September 3, 2014), 35–36, accessed February 27, 2019. doi:10.1177/1529100614546119.

Chapter 7: Habit #1 Nutrient Load – Am I Malnourished?

1. Stacy Simon, "World Health Organization Says Processed Meat Causes Cancer," American Cancer Society, October 26, 2015, accessed January 27, 2019, *https://www.cancer.org/latest-news/world-health-organization-says-processed-meat-causes-cancer.html*.

2. Federation of American Societies for Experimental Biology (FASEB), "Highly Processed Foods Dominate U. S. Grocery Purchases," Science Daily, March 29, 2015, accessed January 20, 2019, *http://www.sciencedaily.com/releases/2015/03/150329141017.htm*.

3. Agence France-Presse, "Unhealthy Eating Linked To 400,000 US Deaths Per Year: Study," NDTV, March 10, 2017, accessed January 20, 2019, *https://www.ndtv.com/health/unhealthy-eating-linked-to-400-000-us-deaths-per-year-study-1668102*.

4. Kimberly Hartke, "Violent Behavior Linked to Nutritional Deficiencies," *Well Being Journal*, January/February 2014, 33–34.

5. Ocean Roberts, "The Anti-Cancer Powerhouses," *What Doctors Don't Tell You: Helping You Make Better Health Choices*, March 2019, 44–53.

6. "Dying for a Burger?" *Nutrition Action Healthletter*, July/August 2017, 7.

7. Ibid.

8. Elizabeth Lipski, *Digestive Wellness*, 3rd ed. (New York: McGraw Hill, 2005), 24.

9. Michael Via, "The Malnutrition of Obesity: Micronutrient Deficiencies That Promote Diabetes," *ISRN Endocrinology* 2012 (January 05, 2012): 1–8, doi:10.5402/2012/103472.

10. Jayson Calton and Mira Calton, The Micronutrient Miracle: The 28-day Plan to Lose Weight, Increase Your Energy, and Reverse Disease (Melbourne, Victoria.: Black Books, 2016), 26.

11. Michael Greger and Gene Stone, How Not to Die: Discover the Foods Scientifically Proven to Prevent and Reverse Disease (London: Pan Books, 2018).

12. Ibid.

13. Sarah Gottfried, The Hormone Cure: Reclaim Balance, Sleep, Sex Drive, and Vitality Naturally with the Gottfried Protocol (New York: Scribner, 2013).

14. Lisa Oz, "The Oz Rx: Eat for a Long Life," *Dr. Oz: The Good Life*, 2017, 66.

15. Carolyn Costin, *The Eating Disorders Sourcebook 3rd ed.* (New York: McGraw-Hill, 2007), 224.

16. Arne Astrup and Susanne Bügel, "Overfed but Undernourished: Recognizing Nutritional Inadequacies/Deficiencies in Patients with Overweight or Obesity," *International Journal of Obesity* 43, no. 2 (July 06, 2018): 219–232, accessed March 03, 2019, doi:10.1038/s41366-018-0143-9.

17. Jayson Calton and Mira Calton, "Obesity and Its Connection to Micronutrient Deficiency – the Evidence Is Becoming Stronger," Calton Nutrition, September 29, 2015, accessed January 08, 2019, *https://www.caltonnutrition.com/obesity-and-micronutrient-deficiency/*.

18. Donald R. Davis, Melvin D. Epp, and Hugh D. Riordan, "Changes in USDA Food Composition Data for 43 Garden Crops, 1950 to 1999," *Journal of the American College of Nutrition* 23, no. 6 (May 07, 2004): 669–682, doi:10.1080/07315724.2004.10719409.

19. Ibid.

20. Calton and Calton, "Obesity and Its Connection to Micronutrient Deficiency – the Evidence Is Becoming Stronger."

21. Astrup and S. Bügel, "Micronutrient Deficiency in the Aetiology of Obesity," *International Journal of Obesity* 34, no. 6 (2010): 947–948, doi:10.1038/ijo.2010.81.

22. Michael Moss, *Salt, Sugar, Fat How the Food Giants Hooked Us* (London: WH Allen, 2014), 42.

23. Ibid.

24. Joseph Mercola and James DiNicolantonio, "The Healthy Brain: Fattening Up the Brain," *What Doctors Don't Tell You: Helping You Make Better Health Choices*, February 2019, 44–49.

25. *What the Health*, directed by Kip Anderson and Keegan Kuhn, performed by Kip Anderson, Garth Davis, and Dr. Neal Bernard, What the Health, 2017, accessed September 01, 2018, *https://www.amazon.com/*.

26. Ibid.

27. Calton and Calton, The Micronutrient Miracle, 90.

28. Fox News, "Survey Shows 74 Percent of Americans Living with GI Discomfort," Fox News, November 24, 2013, accessed March 08, 2019, *https://www.foxnews.com/health/survey-shows-74-percent-of-americans-living-with-gi-discomfort*.

29. Lipski, *Digestive Wellness*, 23–24.

30. Cate Montana, "Magic Bullets," What Doctors Don't Tell You: Helping You Make Better Health Choices, May 2018, 58–64.

31. Josh Axe, "7 Signs and Symptoms You Have Leaky Gut," Dr. Axe, May 08, 2018, accessed March 08, 2019, *https://draxe. com/7-signs-symptoms-you-have-leaky-gut/*.

32. Julie Malacoff, "The Surprising Way Your Brain and Gut Are Connected – Shape Magazine," Amare Blog, December 21, 2017, accessed March 08, 2019, *http://blog.amare.com/ the-surprising-way-your-brain-and-gut-are-connected-shape-magazine/*.

33. Ibid.

34. Josh Axe, "Leaky Gut Diet and Treatment Plan, Including Top Gut Foods," Dr. Axe, July 30, 2018, accessed March 08, 2019, *https://draxe. com/leaky-gut-diet-treatment/*.

35. Ibid.

36. Josh Axe, "7 Signs and Symptoms You Have Leaky Gut."

37. Edward Group, "The Ultimate Candida Diet Program," Dr. Group's Healthy Living Articles, November 09, 2017, accessed March 08, 2019, *https://www.globalhealingcenter.com/natural-health/ultimate-candida-diet-program/?msclkid=4460dc92d02213d8c68b8010700e5693& utm_source=bing&utm_medium=cpc&utm_campaign=Mycozil NB Blog - Search&utm_term= candida fats&utm_content=Mycozil Candida Diet Avoid NB Blog*.

38. Ibid.

39. Laura Paris and Garland Oka, "SIBO Is the New Candida," Laura Paris, February 27, 2017, accessed March 09, 2019, *https://www. parishealingarts.com/sibo-new-candida/*.

40. William Davis, Wheat Belly: Lose the Wheat, Lose the Weight, and Find Your Path Back to Health (London: Harper Thorsons, 2015), 25.

41. Davis, *Wheat Belly*, 25.

42. Ibid.

43. John Douillard, "5 Things You Never Knew About Gluten . . . But Should," John Douillard's LifeSpa, September 24, 2016, accessed March 08, 2019, *https://lifespa.com/5-things-never-knew-gluten-but-should/*.

44. William Davis, Wheat Belly Slim Guide: The Fast and Easy Reference for Living and Succeeding on the Wheat Belly Lifestyle (Emmaus, PA: Rodale, 2017), 4.

45. Davis, *Wheat Belly*, 70.

46. John Douillard, "Do Low-Gluten Diets Increase Type 2 Diabetes Risk?" John Douillard's LifeSpa, May 31, 2017, accessed March 08, 2019, *https://lifespa.com/do-low-gluten-diets-increase-type-2-diabetes-risk/*.

47. Yoko Watanabe et al., "Skipping Breakfast Is Correlated with Obesity," *Journal of Rural Medicine* 9, no. 2 (June 17, 2014): 51–58, doi:10.2185/jrm.2887.

48. Sid Kirchheimer, "Breakfast Reduces Diabetes, Heart Disease," WebMD, March 06, 2003, accessed March 08, 2019, *https://www.webmd.com/diabetes/news/20030306/breakfast-reduces-diabetes-heart-disease#1*.

49. Greger and Stone, *How Not to Die*, 157.

50. Diana Kelly, "21 Ways to Lose a Pound a Week," *The Complete Guide to Diets That Work* (New York: Centennial Living Media, 2018), 20–23.

Chapter 8: Habit #2 Cleanse – Am I Toxic?

1. Lindsay Wilson, *Genetically-Modified Foods: Your Right to Know* (Lakewood, CO: Natural Grocers, 2013).

2. "Man: The Chemical Ape," *nursingschoolhub.com*, accessed January 11, 2019, *https://www.nursingschoolhub.com/chemical-ape/*.

3. Ibid.

4. David Schardt, "Kicking the Can: When Food Containers Become Part of Your Meal," *Nutrition Action Healthletter*, November 2017, 8–11.

5. David Schardt, "Safe at the Plate," *Nutrition Action*, December 2017, 3–6.

6. "Parasites – Toxoplasmosis (Toxoplasma Infection)," Centers for Disease Control and Prevention, October 02, 2018, accessed March 02, 2019, *https://www.cdc.gov/parasites/toxoplasmosis/gen_info/faqs.html*.

7. Joseph Hattersley, "How Chlorine Is Detrimental in Our Water," *Well Being Journal*, May/June 2006, 18–24.

8. Lindsay Wilson, Trust Us, It's Harmless: Could the Popular Herbicide Glyphosate Be Destroying Our Health? (Lakewood, CO: Natural Grocers, 2015).

9. Ibid.

10. Lynne McTaggart and Bryan Hubbard, "Cell Phone Radiation Could Explain Diplomats' Mysterious Illness," *What Doctors Don't Tell You: Helping You Make Better Health Choices*, January 15, 2019.

11. "The Problem with Parabens," What Doctors Don't Tell You: Helping You Make Better Health Choices, February 2019, 72–73.

12. Don Colbert, MD, Toxic Relief: Restore Health and Energy through Fasting and Detoxification (Lake Mary, FL: Siloam, 2012).

13. "Colon Cancer Facts," Colon Cancer Coalition, accessed March 02, 2019, *https://coloncancercoalition.org/get-educated/what-you-need-to-know/colon-cancer-facts/*.

14. Ibid.

15. Karol K. Truman, *Feelings Buried Alive Never Die* (Phoenix: Olympus Publishing Company, 2003), 238.

16. Anna Medaris Miller, "8 Myths about Constipation," *U.S. News & World Report*, April 05, 2015, accessed January 25, 2019, *https://health.usnews.com/health-news/health-wellness/articles/2015/04/08/8-myths-about-constipation*.

17. Diane Quagliani and Patricia Felt-Gunderson, "Closing America's Fiber Intake Gap," *American Journal of Lifestyle Medicine* 11, no. 1 (July 07, 2016): 80–85, doi:10.1177/1559827615588079.

18. Ibid.

19. Quagliani and Gunderson, "Closing America's Fiber Intake Gap."

20. Jess White, "Going with the Gut," *Psychology Today*, July/August 2016, 34–38.

21. Elizabeth Lipski, *Digestive Wellness* (New York: McGraw Hill, 2006), 34.

22. Ibid.

23. Hulda Regehr Clark, *The Cure for All Diseases* (Chula Vista, CA: New Century Press, 1995), 45.

24. Ibid.

25. Ibid.

26. Lyle J. Palmer et al., "Ascaris Lumbricoides Infection Is Associated with Increased Risk of Childhood Asthma and Atopy in Rural China," *American Journal of Respiratory and Critical Care Medicine* 165, no. 11 (January 15, 2002): 1489–1493, accessed January 25, 2019, doi:10.1164/rccm.2107020.

27. Anthony William, Medical Medium Liver Rescue: Answers to Eczema, Psoriasis, Diabetes, Strep, Acne, Gout, Bloating, Gallstones, Adrenal Stress, Fatigue, Fatty Liver, Weight Issues, SIBO, and Autoimmune Disease (Carlsbad, CA: Hay House, 2018), 47.

28. Ibid.

29. Kelsey Casselbury, "The Average Fat Intake in SAD," SF Gate, November 19, 2018, accessed March 04, 2019, *https://healthyeating. sfgate.com/average-fat-intake-sad-11370.html.*

30. VegSource, "What the Dairy Industry Doesn't Want You to Know – Neal Barnard, MD," YouTube, January 28, 2017, accessed March 02, 2019, *https://www.youtube.com/watch?v=h3c_D0s391Q.*

31. Mayo Clinic, "Nearly 7 in 10 Americans Are on Prescription Drugs," *Science Daily,* June 19, 2013, accessed February 19, 2019, *http://www. sciencedaily.com/releases/2013/06/130619132352.htm.*

32. William, *Liver Flush,* 82.

33. Clark, The Cure for All Diseases, 553

34. Truman, Feelings Buried Alive Never Die, 256.

35. Hulda Clark, "Cleanse Flowchart" digital image, Self Health Resource Center, accessed January 15, 2019, *https://drclarkstore.com/ dr-hulda-clark-kidney-cleanse-vegetarian/.*

36. Ibid.

37. Clark, The Cure for All Diseases, 416.

38. Ibid, 417.

Chapter 9: Habit #3 Hydrate – Am I Thirsty?

1. F. Batmanghelidj, Your Body's Many Cries for Water: You're Not Sick; You're Thirsty: Don't Treat Thirst with Medications, Global Health Solutions, 2008, 6.

2. Ibid, 71.

3. Batmanghelidj, Obesity, Cancer, Depression: Their Common Cause & Natural Cure (Falls Church, VA: Global Health Solutions, 2005), 117.

4. Jessica Cerretani, "Water & Health," Whole Living: Body Soul, July/ August 2008, 94–99.

5. Jayne Leonard, "How Often Should You Pee? What's Normal and What's Perfect?" Medical News Today, April 11, 2018, accessed March 04, 2019, *https://www.medicalnewstoday.com/articles/321461.php.*

6. "5 Steps to Fewer Kidney Stones," Nutrition Action, October 2017, 7.

7. Ibid.

8. Ibid.

9. Caitlin Dow, "Low-Cal Sweeteners," Nutrition Action, September 2017, 7–9.

10. Ibid.

11. Ibid, 32.

12. University Saarland. "Blood is thicker than water – and blood plasma is, too," Science Daily, accessed March 13, 2019, *www.sciencedaily.com/releases/2013/02/130218092505.htm.*

13. Batmanghelidj, Obesity, Cancer, Depression: Their Common Cause & Natural Cure, 36.

14. Kerry Brandis, "Fluid Physiology," Fluid Physiology: 2.1 Fluid Compartments, accessed March 04, 2019, *https://www.anaesthesiamcq.com/FluidBook/fl2_1.php.*

15. Mary C. White et al., "Age and Cancer Risk," American Journal of Preventive Medicine 46, no. 3 (March 2014): S7–S15, accessed March 13, 2019, doi:10.1016/j.amepre.2013.10.029.

16. Batmanghelidj, Your Body's Many Cries for Water, 75.

17. Ibid.

18. Kristen Dold, "Healthy-Up Your Blood Pressure," Dr. Oz: The Good Life, 2017, 16–17.

19. Batmanghelidj, Obesity, Cancer, Depression: Their Common Cause & Natural Cure, 171–175.

20. Russell Mariani, "Watercure for a Healthy Body," Well Being Journal, 2014, 22–24.

21. Ibid.

22. Nicholas Bakalar,"37.2 Trillion: Galaxies or Human Cells?" New York Times, June 19, 2015, accessed March 20, 2019, *https://www.nytimes.com/2015/06/23/science/37-2-trillion-galaxies-or-human-cells.html*

23. Mayo Clinic Staff, "Water: How Much Should You Drink Every Day?" Mayo Clinic, September 06, 2017, accessed January 27, 2019, *https://www.mayoclinic.org/healthy-lifestyle/nutrition-and-healthy-eating/in-depth/water/art-20044256.*

24. "Facts on Health Risks of Sugar Drinks," Center for Science in the Public Interest, January 17, 2017, accessed January 28, 2017, *cspinet.org/resource/facts-health-risks-sugar-drinks.*

25. Ibid.

26. Ibid.

27. Isabelle Z., "Pepsi Admits Its Soda Contains Cancer-Causing Ingredients," Natural News, September 15, 2016, accessed March 14, 2019, *https:// www.naturalnews.com/055309_Pepsi_carcinogens_4-Mel.html.*

28. Diana Kelly, "21 Ways to Lose a Pound a Week," The Complete Guide to Diets That Work (New York: Centennial Living Media, LLC, 2018), 20–23.

29. Melonie Heron, "Deaths: Leading Causes for 2016," National Vital Statistics Reports, July 26, 2018, 1–77.

30. Batmanghelidj, Your Body's Many Cries for Water, 103–106.

31. Ibid.

32. Ibid.

33. Thomas Foechlich, "7 Drinks That May Affect Your Cancer Risk," UT Southwestern Medical Center, June 29, 2016, accessed March 13, 2019, *https://utswmed.org/medblog/energy-drink-alcohol-cancer/.*

34. Mayo Clinic Staff, "Water: How Much Should You Drink Every Day?" Mayo Clinic, Mayo Foundation for Medical Education and Research, September 06, 2017, accessed January 27, 2019, *www.mayoclinic.org/ healthy-lifestyle/nutrition-and-healthy-eating/in-depth/water/art-20044 256.*

35. Batmanghelidj, Your Body's Many Cries for Water, 135.

36. Ibid.

37. Batmanghelidj, Your Body's Many Cries for Water, 157–159.

Chapter 10: Habit #4 Sleep – Am I Tired?

1. Bonnie Liebman, "Short on Sleep," Nutrition Action Healthletter, June 2017, 8–9.

2. Ibid.

3. Shawn Stevenson, Sleep Smarter: 21 Essential Strategies to Sleep Your Way to a Better Body, Better Health, and Bigger Success (New York: Rodale Books, 2016), 51.

4. Diana Kelly, "21 Ways to Lose a Pound a Week," The Complete Guide to Diets That Work (New York: Centennial Living Media, LLC, 2018) 20–23.

5. Stevenson, Sleep Smarter, 51.

6.   Kelly, "21 Ways to Lose a Pound a Week."

7.   Alexandros N. Vgontzas et al., "Obesity and Self-Reported Short Sleep Duration: A Marker of Sleep Complaints and Chronic Psychosocial Stress," Sleep Medicine Clinics 4, no. 1 (2009): 65–75, accessed April 24, 2018, doi:10.1016/j.jsmc.2009.01.001.

8.   Ibid.

9.   Ibid.

10. Sara Gottfried, The Hormone Cure: Reclaim Balance, Sleep, Sex Drive, and Vitality Naturally with the Gottfried Protocol (New York: Scribner, 2013) 101.

11. Liebman, "Short on Sleep," Nutrition Action Healthletter, 8–9.

12. Brian Tefft, "Asleep at the Wheel: The Prevalence of Drowsy Driving," November 2010, accessed March 4, 2019, *http://www.greylit.org/sites/ default/files/collected_files/2012-12/2010DrowsyDrivingReport_1.pdf.*

13. Shawn Stevenson, Sleep Smarter, 111.

14. "Americans Are Getting More ZZZZs," Penn Medicine News, January 18, 2018, accessed March 04, 2019, *https://www.pennmedicine.org/news/ news-releases/2018/january/americans-are-getting-more-zzzzs.*

15. Vgontzas et al., "Obesity and Self-Reported Short Sleep Duration: A Marker of Sleep Complaints and Chronic Psychosocial Stress."

16. Liebman, "Short on Sleep," Nutrition Action Healthletter, 8–9.

17. M. Williamson and Anne-Marie Feyer, "Moderate Sleep Deprivation Produces Impairments in Cognitive and Motor Performance Equivalent to Legally Prescribed Levels of Alcohol Intoxication," Occupational and Environmental Medicine 57, no. 10 (2000): 649–655, accessed January 31, 2019, *oem.bmj.com/content/oemed/57/10/649.full.pdf.*

18. Stevenson, Sleep Smarter, 105.

19. Vgontzas et al., "Obesity and Self-Reported Short Sleep Duration: A Marker of Sleep Complaints and Chronic Psychosocial Stress."

20. Teresa Arora et al., "The Impact of Sleep Debt on Excess Adiposity and Insulin Sensitivity in Patients with Early Type 2 Diabetes Mellitus," Journal of Clinical Sleep Medicine 12, no. 05 (May 15, 2016): 673–680, accessed February 11, 2019, doi:10.5664/jcsm.5792.

21. Vgontzas et al., "Obesity and Self-Reported Short Sleep Duration: A Marker of Sleep Complaints and Chronic Psychosocial Stress."

22. Liebman, "Short on Sleep," Nutrition Action Healthletter, 8–9.

23. Shahrad Taheri et al., "Short Sleep Duration Is Associated with Reduced Leptin, Elevated Ghrelin, and Increased Body Mass Index," PLoS Medicine 1, no. 3 (December 07, 2004), accessed January 31, 2019, doi: 10.1371/journal.pmed.0010062.

24. Liebman, "Short on Sleep," Nutrition Action Healthletter, 8–9.

25. Celeste McGovern, "Smash Your Addictions," What Doctors Don't Tell You: Helping You Make Better Health Choices, May 2018, 28–37.

26. Ibid.

27. Proceedings of the European Society of Cardiology Congress, Munich, Germany, August 26, 2018, ed. "Sleep Sweet Spot Is Six to Eight Hours a Day," What Doctors Don't Tell You: Helping You Make Better Health Choices, January 2019, 12.

28. Hulda Regehr Clark, The Cure for All Diseases (Chula Vista, CA: New Century Press, 1995), 244.

29. Helen Messina, "Detoxifiers for High Ammonia Levels Due to Liver Diseases," Livestrong, accessed March 04, 2019, *https://www.livestrong.com/article/351568-detoxifiers-for-high-ammonia-levels-due-to-liver-diseases/.*

30. Clark, The Cure for All Diseases, 244.

31. Ann Miller-Cohen, "The Art of Cooking Green Gourmet Foods," Well Being Journal, May/June 2006, 14–18.

32. Fumito Naganuma et al., "Histamine N-methyltransferase Regulates Aggression and the Sleep-wake Cycle," Scientific Reports 7, no. 1 (November 21, 2017), doi:10.1038/s41598-017-16019-8.

33. Stephen Cherniske, Caffeine Blues: Wake up to the Hidden Dangers of Americas #1 Drug (New York: Warner, 1998), 98.

34. Ibid.

35. Pauline Harding, "Eat Your Way to Better Sleep," Well Being Journal, March/April 2008, 5–10.

36. Ibid.

37. "Curb Carbs at Dinner," Nutrition Action Healthletter, May 2017, 8.

38. Harding, "Eat Your Way to Better Sleep," 5–10.

39. Ibid.

40. Jason Fung, The Obesity Code: Unlocking the Secrets of Weight Loss (Vancouver: Greystone Books, 2016), 94.

41. Ibid.

42. Pauline Harding, "Eat Your Way to Better Sleep," 5–10.

43. Sara Gottfried, The Hormone Cure,134.

44. Abbasi et al., "The Effect of Magnesium Supplementation on Primary Insomnia in Elderly: A Double-blind Placebo-controlled Clinical Trial," Current Neurology and Neuroscience Reports, December 17, 2012, accessed March 06, 2019, *https://www.ncbi.nlm.nih.gov/pubmed/23853635*.

45. Michael J. Breus, "Magnesium – How It Affects Your Sleep," Psychology Today, May 2, 2018, accessed March 06, 2019, *https://www.psychologytoday.com/us/blog/sleep-newzzz/201805/magnesium-how-it-affects-your-sleep*.

46. Chris Gilbert, "Repressed Emotions and Physical Illness," Well Being Journal, April/May 2018, 20–23.

47. Liebman, "Short on Sleep," Nutrition Action Healthletter, 8–9.

48. Sara Gottfried, The Hormone Cure, 101.

49. Vyga Kaufmann, TEDx Talks, YouTube, October 22, 2015, accessed January 05, 2019, *https://www.youtube.com/watch?v=WNj1Y11t_x8*.

50. Ibid.

51. Dave Asprey, "Bulletproof Your Sleep with vitamin D | When to Take vitamin D," Bulletproof, June 04, 2018, accessed January 27, 2019, *https://blog.bulletproof.com/bulletproof-your-sleep-with-vitamin-d/#ref-5*.

52. Michael Breus, "The Latest on Blue Light and Sleep," The Sleep Doctor: Your Guide to Better Sleep, November 06, 2017, accessed March 06, 2019, *https://thesleepdoctor.com/2017/11/06/latest-blue-light-sleep/*.

53. Borge Sivertsen et al., "Use of Sleep Medications and Mortality: The Hordaland Health Study," Drugs – Real World Outcomes 2, no. 2 (May 05, 2015): 123–128, doi:10.1007/s40801-015-0023-8.

54. Ibid.

Chapter 11: Habit #4 Exercise – Am I Inactive?

1. Steven C. Moore et al., "Association of Leisure-Time Physical Activity with Risk of 26 Types of Cancer in 1.44 Million Adults," *JAMA Internal Medicine* 176, no. 6 (June 01, 2016): 816–25, doi:10.1001/jamainternmed.2016.1548.

2. Alexandra Sifferlin, "The Truth about Running," *The Science of Exercise, Special ed.* (New York: Time Books, Inc., 2017), 68–69.

3. Dr. Mercola, "The Right Dose of Exercise for a Longer Life," mercola. com, accessed January 02, 2019, *https://fitness.mercola.com/sites/fitness/ archive/2015/05/01/right-dose-exercise-for-long-life.aspx*.

4. Dr. Mercola, "How Short Bursts of Exercise Help Decrease Disease and Risk of Death," mercola.com, April 6, 2018, accessed March 06, 2019, *https://fitness.mercola.com/sites/fitness/archive/2018/04/06/short-bursts- exercise-may-prevent-death.aspx*.

5. Sifferlin, "The Truth about Running," 68–69.

6. Many Oaklander, "The Power of Strength Training," *The Science of Exercise, Special ed.* (New York: Time Books, Inc., 2017), 40–45.

7. Oaklander, "The Power of Strength Training," 40–45.

8. Alyssa Shaffer, "The Truth about Weight Loss," *The Science of Exercise* Special ed. (New York: Time Books, Inc., 2017), 36–37.

9. Markham Heid, "The Truth about Walking," *The Science of Exercise* Special ed. (New York: Time Books, Inc., 2017), 92–93.

10. Heid, "The Truth about Walking," 92–93.

11. Alexandra Sifferlin, "How to Exercise When You Have No Time," *The Science of Exercise* Special ed. (New York: Time Books, Inc., 2017), 82–85.

12. Ibid.

13. Ibid.

14. Ibid.

15. Caitlin Dow, "Exercise: Can You Trust the Latest Buzz?" *Nutrition Action Healthletter*, April 2017, 9–11.

16. Alice Park, "How Exercise Keeps You Young," *The Science of Exercise, Special ed.* (New York: Time Books, Inc., 2017), 24–27.

17. D. Reimers et al. "Does Physical Activity Increase Life Expectancy? A Review of the Literature," *Journal of Aging Research* 2012, July 1, 2012, 1–9, doi:10.1155/2012/243958.

18. Kristen Dold, "Healthy-Up Your Blood Pressure," *Dr. Oz: The Good Life*, 2017, 16–17.

19. Caitlin Dow, "Exercise: Can You Trust the Latest Buzz?" *Nutrition Action Newsletter*, April 2017, 9–11.

20. Camille Noe Pagan, "The Fitness Rx," *The Science of Exercise* Special ed. (New York: Time Books, Inc., 2017), 18–21.

21. Ibid.

22. Mandy Oaklander, "The Power of Strength Training," *The Science of Exercise* Special ed. (New York: Time Books, Inc., 2017), 40–45.

23. Mandy Oaklander, "The New Science of Exercise," *The Science of Exercise* Special ed. (New York: Time Books, Inc., 2017), 10–17.

24. Jacques Steinberg, "Anyone Can Be an Ironman," *The Science of Exercise* Special ed. (New York: Time Books, Inc., 2017), 86–91.

25. "Physical Activity and Adults," World Health Organization, June 19, 2015, accessed March 05, 2019, *https://www.who.int/dietphysicalactivity/factsheet_adults/en/.*

26. "Reality Bites," *The Complete Guide to Diets That Work* (New York: Centennial Living Media, 2018), 96.

27. Ellie Zolfagharifard, "You Should Be Working Out for More than an Hour a Day, Claim Scientists," Daily Mail Online, April 15, 2015, accessed January 02, 2019, *https://www.dailymail.co.uk/sciencetech/article-3040911/Forget-doing-150-minutes-exercise-week-working-HOUR-day-claim-scientists.html.*

28. Caitlin Dow, "Exercise: Can You Trust the Latest Buzz?" *Nutrition Action Healthletter*, April 2017, 9–11.

29. Diana Kelly, "21 Ways to Lose a Pound a Week," *The Complete Guide to Diets That Work* (New York: Centennial Living Media, 2018), 20–23.

30. Dow, "Exercise: Can You Trust the Latest Buzz?" 9–11.

31. Ibid.

32. Heid, "The Truth about Walking," 92–93.

33. Camille Noe Pagan, "The Fitness Rx," *The Science of Exercise* Special ed. (New York: Time Books, Inc., 2017), 18–21.

34. Park, "How Exercise Keeps You Young," 24–27.

35. Ibid.

36. Oaklander, "The New Science of Exercise," 15.

37. Dow, "Exercise: Can You Trust the Latest Buzz?" 9–11.

38. Oaklander, "The New Science of Exercise," 15.

39. Dow, "Exercise: Can You Trust the Latest Buzz?" 9–11.

40. Kristin J. Homan et al., "Appearance-based Exercise Motivation Moderates the Relationship between Exercise Frequency and Positive Body Image," *Body Image* 11, no. 2 (March 2014): 101–108, doi:10.1016/j.bodyim.2014.01.003.

41. Mandy Oaklander, "7 Ways to Motivate Yourself to Exercise," *The Science of Exercise* Special ed. (New York: Time Books, Inc., 2017), 72–77.

42. James Clear, "How the 'Seinfeld Strategy' Can Help You Stop Procrastinating," Entrepreneur, January 27, 2014, accessed March 05, 2019, *https://www.entrepreneur.com/article/231023*.

43. "Camino De Santiago," Wikipedia, February 25, 2019, accessed March 14, 2019, *https://en.wikipedia.org/wiki/Camino_de_Santiago*.

44. Ibid.

45. Oaklander, "7 Ways to Motivate Yourself to Exercise."

Chapter 12: Habit #6 Balance – Am I Hormonal?

1. Sara Gottfried, The Hormone Cure: Reclaim Balance, Sleep, Sex Drive, and Vitality Naturally with the Gottfried Protocol (New York: Scribner, 2013), 101.

2. Ibid.

3. Gary Donovitz, Age Healthier, Live Happier: Avoiding Over-Medication through Natural Hormone Balance (Orlando: Celebrity Press, 2015), 87.

4. Ibid, 57.

5. Gottfried, *The Hormone Cure*, 46.

6. Gary Taubes, *Why We Get Fat: And What to Do about It* (New York: Anchor Books, 2011), 134.

7. Carina Wolff, "Does Exercising Affect Your Homones? You Might Feel These 8 Changes," Bustle, August 16, 2018, accessed February 19, 2019, *https://www.bustle.com/p/does-exercising-affect-your-hormones-you-might-feel-these-8-changes-10127007*.

8. Gottfried, *The Hormone Cure*, 135.

9. "Sperm Counts on the Decline," *Nutrition Action Healthletter*, November 2017, 3.

10. Mary Shomon, "Why Is Cortisol So Controversial for Weight Loss?" Verywell Health, October 8, 2018, accessed February 11, 2019, *https://www.verywellhealth.com/the-cortisol-weight-loss-controversy-3233036*.

11. Leonardo Trasande, Sicker, Fatter, Poorer: The Urgent Threat of Hormone-Disrupting Chemicals on Our Health and Future ... and What We Can Do about It (Boston: Houghton Mifflin Harcourt, 2019), 139.

12. Juliet Wilkinson, "Are Hormones in Meat Affecting Humans?" Livestrong, accessed March 09, 2019, *https://www.livestrong.com/ article/464430-are-hormones-in-meat-affecting-humans/*.

13. Nick Garcia, "4 Hormone Imbalances Preventing You from Losing Weight," Upgraded Health, January 14, 2019, accessed March 06, 2019, *https://upgradedhealth. net/4-hormone-imbalances-preventing-you-from-losing-weight/*.

14. Gottfried, *The Hormone Cure,* 163.

15. Garcia, "4 Hormone Imbalances Preventing You from Losing Weight."

16. Center for Veterinary Medicine, "Product Safety Information – Steroid Hormone Implants Used for Growth in Food-Producing Animals," US Food and Drug Administration Home Page, accessed March 10, 2019, *https://www.fda.gov/animalveterinary/safetyhealth/productsafetyinformation/ ucm055436.htm*.

17. Juliet Wilkinson, "Are Hormones in Meat Affecting Humans?" Livestrong, accessed March 09, 2019, *https://www.livestrong.com/ article/464430-are-hormones-in-meat-affecting-humans/*.

18. "Recombinant Bovine Growth Hormone," American Cancer Society, September 10, 2014, accessed March 10, 2019, *https://www.cancer.org/ cancer/cancer-causes/recombinant-bovine-growth-hormone.html*.

19. Interview with Vegan Outreach, August 18, 2018, accessed August 18, 2018, *https://www.facebook.com/jendayi.harris/ videos/2225625044133579/*.

20. Carina Storrs, "Hormones in Food: Should You Worry?" Health, October 22, 2011, accessed March 10, 2019, *https://www.health.com/ health/article/0,,20458816,00.html*.

21. "Recombinant Bovine Growth Hormone."

22. "Sperm Counts on the Decline."

23. Juliet Wilkinson, "Are Hormones in Meat Affecting Humans?" Livestrong.com, accessed March 09, 2019, *https://www.livestrong.com/ article/464430-are-hormones-in-meat-affecting-humans/*.

24. Josh Axe, "High-Estrogen Foods to Avoid (Some Mess with Breast Cancer Treatment!)," Dr. Axe, October 15, 2018, accessed February 12, 2019, *https://draxe.com/5-high-estrogen-foods-avoid/*.

25. "The FoodPrint of Beef," FoodPrint, accessed March 10, 2019, *https:// foodprint.org/reports/the-foodprint-of-beef/?cid=258*.

26. Jason Fung, *The Obesity Code: Unlocking the Secrets of Weight Loss* (Vancouver: Greystone Books, 2016), 87.

27. Dr. Jason Fung, "Insulin and Weight Gain – Hormonal Obesity," Intensive Dietary Management (IDM), May 26, 2018, accessed March 09, 2019, *https://idmprogram.com/ insulin-causes-weight-gain-hormonal-obesity-iv/*.

28. Laura Dolson, "Insulin Resistance Symptoms, Causes, and Treatment," Very Well Health, January 03, 2019, accessed February 7, 2019, *https:// www.verywellhealth.com/what-is-insulin-resistance-2242260*.

29. Integrated Diabetes Services, Gary Scheiner, "Insulin & Weight Gain: Does Tighter Control Make You Loosen Your Belt?" Diabetes Strong, January 20, 2018, accessed February 10, 2019, *https://diabetesstrong.com/ insulin-weight-gain-does-tighter-control-make-you-loosen-your-belt/*.

30. Fung, "Insulin and Weight Gain – Hormonal Obesity."

31. Fung, *The Obesity Code*, 175.

32. Franziska Spritzler, "12 Natural Ways to Balance Your Hormones." Healthline, May 15, 2017, accessed February 12, 2019, *https://www. healthline.com/nutrition/balance-hormones#section12*.

33. Taubes, *Why We Get Fat*, 90–95,105.

34. Ibid, 136–139.

35. D. Anton et al., "Flipping the Metabolic Switch: Understanding and Applying the Health Benefits of Fasting," *Obesity* 26, no. 2 (October 31, 2017): 254–268, doi:10.1002/oby.22065.

36. Hiliary Parker, "A Sweet Problem: Princeton Researchers Find That High-fructose Corn Syrup Prompts Considerably More Weight Gain," Princeton University, March 22, 2010, accessed March 09, 2019, *https://www.princeton.edu/news/2010/03/22/ sweet-problem-princeton-researchers-find-high-fructose-corn-syrup-prompts*.

37. Fung, *The Obesity Code*, 164.

38. Ibid.

39. Parker, "A Sweet Problem: Princeton Researchers Find That High-Fructose Corn Syrup Prompts Considerably More Weight Gain," 1.

40. Fung, *The Obesity Code*, 246–247.

41. Ibid, 120.

42. D. Anton et al., "Flipping the Metabolic Switch: Understanding and Applying the Health Benefits of Fasting."

43. Fung, The Obesity Code, 92–94.

44. Gottfried, The Hormone Cure, 331.

45. Ibid, 24–25.

46. Ibid, 86.

47. Fung, The Obesity Code, 92.

48. Ibid, 94.

49. Taubes, Why We Get Fat, 124.

50. Dr. Len Lopez, "Stress and Hormone Imbalances," The Christian Post, accessed March 09, 2019, https://www.christianpost.com/news/stress-and-hormone-imbalances.html.

51. Josh Axe, "Adrenal Fatigue Symptoms, Diet & Remedies," Dr. Axe, November 01, 2018, accessed March 08, 2019, https://draxe.com/3-steps-to-heal-adrenal-fatigue/.

52. Dave Korsunsky, "Basal Body Temperature Tracking – Part One – Thyroid," Heads Up Health, September 17, 2017, accessed March 10, 2019, https://www.headsuphealth.com/blog/self-tracking/basal-body-temperature-tracking-part-one-thyroid/.

53. Gottfried, The Hormone Cure, 333.

54. Broda Otto Barnes and Lawrence Galton, Hypothyroidism: The Unsuspected Illness (New York: Harper & Row, 1976), 23–24.

55. Ibid.

56. Dave Korsunsky, "Basal Body Temperature Tracking – Part One – Thyroid."

57. Ibid.

58. N. Walter et al., "Elevated Thyroid Stimulating Hormone Is Associated with Elevated Cortisol in Healthy Young Men and Women," Thyroid Research 5, no. 1 (October 30, 2012): 13, doi:10.1186/1756-6614-5-13.

59. Gottfried, The Hormone Cure, 242.

60. Walter, "Elevated Thyroid Stimulating Hormone Is Associated with Elevated Cortisol in Healthy Young Men and Women."

61. Jacqueline Jacques, "The Role of Your Thyroid in Metabolism and Weight Control," Obesity Action Coalition, accessed March 09, 2019, https://www.obesityaction.org/community/article-library/the-role-of-your-thyroid-in-metabolism-and-weight-control/.

62. American Thyroid Association, "Thyroid and Weight," American Thyroid Association, accessed March 09, 2019, *https://www.thyroid.org/thyroid-and-weight/.*

63. Ibid.

64. Anthony William, Medical Medium Thyroid Healing: The Truth behind Hashimotos, Graves, Insomnia, Hypothyroidism, Thyroid Nodules & Epstein-Barr (Carlsbad, CA: Hay House, 2017), 29.

65. Anthony William, "Epstein Barr Virus Revealed," Medical Medium, accessed March 9, 2019, *http://www.medicalmedium.com/blog/epstein-barr-virus-revealed.*

66. William, *Thyroid Healing*, 99.

67. Dana Trentini, "Hypothyroidism Symptoms," Hypothyroid Mom, accessed February 12, 2019, *https://hypothyroidmom.com/category/hypothyroidism-symptoms/.*

68. Ibid.

69. Ibid.

70. Izabela Wentz, "Fluoride and Your Thyroid," Thyroid Pharmacist, March 15, 2018, accessed March 10, 2019, *https://thyroidpharmacist.com/articles/fluoride-and-your-thyroid/.*

71. Anna Cabeca, "What Men Need to Know about Healthy Testosterone Levels," Dr. Anna Cabeca, date written, accessed February 12, 2019, *https://drannacabeca.com/blogs/mens-health/what-men-need-to-know-about-healthy-testosterone-levels.*

72. Ibid.

73. Mary Elizabeth Dallas, "The Link Between Low Testosterone and Diabetes," Stroke Center – Everyday Health, January 16, 2014, accessed February 12, 2019, *https://www.everydayhealth.com/hs/low-testosterone-guide/low-testosterone-diabetes/.*

74. Ibid.

75. Gottfried, *The Hormone Cure*, 345.

76. Anna Cabeca, "What Men Need to Know about Healthy Testosterone Levels."

77. Donovitz, Age Healthier Live Happier, 87.

78. Gottfried, *The Hormone Cure*, 182.

79. Andre Harris, TEDx Talks, YouTube, December 05,
     2018, accessed January 2, 2019. *https://www.youtube.com/
     watch?time_continue=1&v=ZiDfZLJZTGU.*

80. Jade Teta, "Female Hormones: Estrogen (Oestrogen) & Weight Loss,"
     Metabolic Effect, June 10, 2013, accessed February 11, 2019, *https://
     www.metaboliceffect.com/female-hormones-estrogen/.*

81. Axe, "High-Estrogen Foods to Avoid."

82. Taubes, *Why We Get Fat*, 90.

83. Laura Paris and Anita Sadaty. "4 Causes of Hormone Imbalance
     and 5 Ways to Fix It," My Hormone Answers, January 18,
     2019, accessed March 11, 2019, *https://myhormoneanswers.
     com/4-causes-of-hormone-imbalance-and-5-ways-to-fix-it/.*

84. Debra Rose Wilson, "Signs and Symptoms of High Estrogen,"
     Healthline, February 20, 2018, accessed February 7, 2019, *https://www.
     healthline.com/health/high-estrogen#outlook.*

85. Gottfried, *The Hormone Cure*, 163.

86. Cabeca, "What Men Need to Know about Healthy Testosterone Levels."

87. Gottfried, *The Hormone Cure*, 27.

88. Wilson, "Signs and Symptoms of High Estrogen."

89. Marion Gluck, "Estrogen Dominance and Hypothyroidism," Marion
     Gluck Clinic, April 23, 2018, accessed February 12, 2019, *https://www.
     mariongluckclinic.com/blog/estrogen-dominance-hypothyroidism.html.*

90. Carrie Drzyzga, "Signs of Estrogen Deficiency," The Functional
     Medicine Radio Show with Dr. Carrie, February 24, 2016, accessed
     March 11, 2019, *https://www.drcarri.com/signs-of-estrogen-deficiency/.*

91. James, "High Estrogen vs. Low Estrogen Symptoms (For Men),"
     Dosage May Vary, August 23, 2017, accessed February 11, 2019, *https://
     dosagemayvary.com/high-estrogen-vs-low-estrogen-symptoms-for-men/.*

92. Drzyzga, "Signs of Estrogen Deficiency."

93. Gottfried, *The Hormone Cure*, 179.

94. Ibid.

95. Taubes, *Why We Get Fat*, 90.

96. Ibid.

97. Wilson, "Signs and Symptoms of High Estrogen."

98. Gottfried, *The Hormone Cure*, 345.

99.   Taubes, *Why We Get Fat*, 90.

100. Lindsay Wilson. *Genetically-Modified Foods: Your Right to Know* (Lakewood, CO: Natural Grocers, 2013).

101. Natural News. "'Most Thorough Research' to Date Links GMO Corn to Tumors, Organ Damage, and Premature Death in Rats," Food Matters®, July 12, 2018, accessed March 10, 2019, *https://www.foodmatters.com/article/gm-corn-linked-to-cancer-tumors*.

102. Axe, "High-Estrogen Foods to Avoid."

103. Ibid.

104. Josh Axe, "How to Balance Hormones Naturally," Dr. Axe, February 04, 2019, accessed March 07, 2019, *https://draxe.com/10-ways-balance-hormones-naturally/)*.

105. Donovitz, Age Healthier Live Happier, 132–133.

106. Aaron Kandola, "10 Health Benefits of Maca Root," Medical News Today, July 18, 2018, accessed February 11, 2019, *https://www.medicalnewstoday.com/articles/322511.php*.

107. The Maca Team, "What Is Maca," The Maca Team, LLC, accessed March 10, 2019, *https://www.themacateam.com/what-is-maca*.

108. Axe, "How to Balance Hormones Naturally."

109. Carina Wolff, "Does Exercising Affect Your Hormones? You Might Feel These 8 Changes," Bustle, August 16, 2018, accessed February 18, 2019, *https://www.bustle.com/p/does-exercising-affect-your-hormones-you-might-feel-these-8-changes-10127007*.

110. Ibid.

111. Women's Health, "PMS," Women's Health, March 16, 2018, accessed March 10, 2019, *https://www.womenshealth.gov/menstrual-cycle/premenstrual-syndrome*.

Chapter 13: Prioritize Body Care

1.   Nadine Roberts Cornish, *Tears in My Gumbo*, Book 1 (Denver: Caregivers Guardian Publishing House, 2017), 6.

2.   Dwayne Johnson, "Dwayne Johnson's Insane Diet and Workouts That Make Him Ripped," YouTube, October 30, 2018, accessed March 09, 2019, *https://www.youtube.com/watch?v=xkY45e5k9sw*.

Chapter 14: Grubbology – Say Hello to Your Inner Glutton

1. Chris Isidore and Tami Luhby, "Turns out Americans Work Really Hard ... but Some Want to Work Harder," CNNMoney, Cable News Network, July 9, 2015, *http://money.cnn.com/2015/07/09/news/economy/americans-work-bush/index.html.*

2. John Bradshaw, *Healing the Shame That Binds You* (Deerfield Beach, FL: Health Communications, Inc., 2005).

3. Mark E. Koltko-Rivera, "Rediscovering the Later Version of Maslows Hierarchy of Needs: Self-Transcendence and Opportunities for Theory, Research, and Unification," *Review of General Psychology* 10 (4) (2006): 302–317, https://doi.org/10.1037/1089-2680.10.4.302.

4. Ibid.

Chapter 15: The Fear of the Whole Self

1. "Torment," Merriam-Webster, *www.merriam-webster.com/dictionary/torment, accessed March 19, 2019.*

2. Marianne Williamson, A Return to Love: Reflections on the Principles of a Course in Miracles (New York: HarperOne, 2012).

3. Pastor Chad Dedmon, BridgeWay Church Denver, YouTube, January 21, 2018, *https://www.youtube.com/watch?v=kHWeCLPhLuA&t=3s.*

4. John Bradshaw, *Healing the Shame That Binds You* (Deerfield Beach, FL: Health Communications, Inc., 2005).

5. Cancer Treatment Centers of America, "More New Cancer Cases Linked to Obesity," Cancers Treatment Center of America, accessed July 1, 2018, *https://www.cancercenter.com/.*

Chapter 16: Chubbology – Why We Self Protect with Weight

1. Child Sexual Abuse Statistics, National Center for Victims of Crime, accessed March 21, 2019, *http://victimsofcrime.org/media/reporting-on-child-sexual-abuse/child-sexual-abuse-statistics.*

2. Olga Khazan, "Abused as Children, Obese as Adults," *The Atlantic,* Atlantic Media Company, December 15, 2015, *https://www.theatlantic.com/health/archive/2015/12/sexual-abuse-victims-obesity/420186/.*

3. Amber Smith, "Experts See Strong Link between Sexual Abuse and Obesity," syracuse.com, July 25, 2010, *https://www.syracuse.com/news/2010/07/linking_sexual_abuse_to_obesit.html.*

4.   Ibid.

5.   Kanaklakshmi Masodkar, Justine Johnson, and Michael J. Peterson, "A Review of Posttraumatic Stress Disorder and Obesity," *The Primary Care Companion for CNS Disorders*, January 2016, *https://doi.org/10.4088/pcc.15r01848.*

6.   Jendayi Harris, "Whole and Free Health Course Survey," The Potter's House Church Denver, June 15, 2018.

7.   "Vulnerable," Merriam-Webster, accessed March 21, 2019, *https://www.merriam-webster.com/dictionary/vulnerable.*

8.   Saul McLeod, "Saul McLeod," Simply Psychology, January 1, 1970. *https://www.simplypsychology.org/self-concept.html.*

9.   Barbra E. Russell, *Yes! I Said No!* (Aurora, CO: Noble House Press, 2017), 23.

Chapter 17: Adopt the Freedom Mindset

1.   "U.S. Weight Loss Market Worth $60.9 Billion," PRWeb, May 9, 2011, *http://www.prweb.com/releases/2011/5/prweb8393658.htm.*

2.   Katherine Schreiber and Diana Kelly, "Don't Fall for It Dietary Fads over the Decades," essay in *The Complete Guide to Diets That Work* (New York: Centennial Living Media, 2018), 20–23.

3.   Ibid, "U.S. Weight Loss Market Worth $60.9 Billion."

4.   Caroline Leaf, Who Switched off My Brain?: Controlling Toxic Thoughts and Emotions (Southlake, TX: Inprov, Ltd., 2009).

5.   Albert Einstein, "Albert Einstein Quotes," BrainyQuote, Xplore, accessed March 19, 2019, *https://www.brainyquote.com/quotes/albert_einstein_121993.*

6.   "How Many Thoughts Do We Have Per Minute?" IAC Publishing, accessed March 25, 2019, *https://www.reference.com/world-view/many-thoughts-per-minute-cb7fcf22ebbf8466.*

7.   Brian Wansink, "Why Dieters Are Doomed on Tuesdays," NBCNews. com, NBCUniversal News Group, May 14, 2007, *http://www.nbcnews.com/id/16472344/ns/health-diet_and_nutrition/t/why-dieters-are-doomed-tuesdays/#.XJi45rhMGUk.*

8.   Sharon Fruh et al., "Meal-Planning Practices with Individuals in Health Disparity Zip Codes." *The Journal for Nurse Practitioners* 9 (6) (2013): 344–349, *https://doi.org/10.1016/j.nurpra.2013.03.016.*

9.   Laura Pratt and Debra Brody, "National Center for Health Statistics," Centers for Disease Control and Prevention, October 16, 2014, *https://www.cdc.gov/nchs/products/databriefs/db167.htm.*

10.   David Engstrom, "Obesity and Depression," Obesity Action Coalition, accessed March 19, 2019, *https://www.obesityaction.org/community/article-library/obesity-and-depression/.*

11.   Marci Shimoff and Carol Kline, *Happy for No Reason: 7 Steps to Being Happy from the Inside Out* (New York: Atria Paperback, 2013), 36.

Chapter 18: Enact an Emotional Strength Training Plan

1.   "Emotions," Merriam-Webster, accessed March 22, 2019, *https://www.merriamwebster.com/dictionary/emotions.*

2.   Peter Scazzero, Emotionally Healthy Spirituality: It's Impossible to be Spiritually Mature while Remaining Emotionally Immature. (Nashville: Thomas Nelson, 2014), 1.

3.   Robert Plutchik, "Emotion Wheel," ToolsHero, July 18, 2018, *https://www.toolshero.com/psychology/personal-happiness/emotion-wheel-robert-plutchik/.*

4.   Otto Kroeger and Janet M. Thuesen, Type Talk: The 16 Personality Types That Determine How We Live, Love, and Work (New York: Dell Trade Paperbacks, 1998), 70.

5.   Wendy Backlund, *Victorious Emotions* (Redding, CA: Igniting Hope Ministries, 2017), 67.

6.   Scazzero, Emotionally Healthy Spirituality, 24.

7.   Ibid, 25.

8.   "Release," Merriam-Webster, accessed March 22, 2019, *https://www.merriam-webster.com/dictionary/release.*

9.   Peggy A. Hannon et al., "The Soothing Effects of Forgiveness on Victims and Perpetrators Blood Pressure," Personal Relationships 19 (2) (2011): 279–28, https://doi.org/10.1111/j.1475-6811.2011.01356.x.

10.   Mayo Clinic Staff, "Why Is It So Easy to Hold a Grudge?" Mayo Clinic, Mayo Foundation for Medical Education and Research, November 4, 2017, *https://www.mayoclinic.org/healthy-lifestyle/adult-health/in-depth/forgiveness/art-20047692.*

11.   Susan McQuillan, "A New Approach to Weight Loss," *Psychology Today*, Sussex Publishers, October 3, 2016, *https://www.psychologytoday.com/us/blog/cravings/201610/new-approach-weight-loss.*

12. Lucene Wisniewski and Denise D. Ben-Porath, "Dialectical Behavior Therapy and Eating Disorders: The Use of Contingency Management Procedures to Manage Dialectical Dilemmas," American Journal of Psychotherapy 69 (2) (2015): 129–140, *https://doi.org/10.1176/appi.psychotherapy.2015.69.2.129.*

13. Carlos M. Grilo et al., "Cognitive-behavioral therapy, behavioral weight loss, and sequential treatment for obese patients with binge-eating disorder: a randomized controlled trial," Journal of Consulting and Clinical Psychology 79 (5) (2011): 675–685, accessed November 18, 2018, *http://commonweb.unifr.ch/artsdean/pub/gestens/f/as/files/4660/33127_093048.pdf.*

14. Sue Popkess-Vawter, "Holistic Self-Care Model for Permanent Weight Control," Journal of Holistic Nursing 11 (4) (1993): 341–355, *https://doi.org/10.1177/089801019301100404.*

Chapter 19: Looksology – Jump off the Body Shame Train

1. "How Body Image Disturbance Relates to Eating Disorders." Eating Disorder Hope, accessed April 5, 2019, *https://www.eatingdisorderhope.com/information/body-image/how-body-image-relates-to-eating-disorders.*

2. Ibid.

3. Tufan Nayir, Ersin Uskun, Mustafa Volkan Yürekli, Hacer Devran, Ayşe Çelik, and Ramazan Azim Okyay. "Does Body Image Affect Quality of Life?: A Population Based Study." PLOS ONE 11, no. 9 (September 20, 2016). *https://doi.org/10.1371/journal.pone.0163290.*

4. "Body Image," National Eating Disorders Collaboration, accessed March 21, 2021, *https://nedc.com.au/eating-disorders/eating-disorders-explained/body-image/.*

5. Renee Engeln, "An Epidemic of Beauty Sickness," TEDxUConn 2013," YouTube, October 21, 2013, *https://www.youtube.com/watch?v=63XsokRPV_Y.*

6. David Garner, "Body Image in America: Survey Results," Psychology Today, Sussex Publishers, February 1, 1997, *https://www.psychologytoday.com/us/articles/199702/body-image-in-america-survey-results.n.*

7. Ibid.

8. Ibid.

9. Ibid.

10. "Psychology: Body Image Graphic," InfographicNow.com, July 5, 2017, *https://infographicnow.com/psychology-infographics/psychology-body-image-graphic-3/*.

11. David Garner, "Body Image in America: Survey Results," Psychology Today, Sussex Publishers, February 1, 1997, *https://www.psychologytoday.com/us/articles/199702/body-image-in-america-survey-results*.

12. Ibid.

13. Ibid.

14. Tina Kelley, "'Am I Too Fat?" *The New York Times*, April 4, 2004, *https://www.nytimes.com/2004/04/04/nyregion/am-i-too-fat.html*.

15. Norwegian University of Science and Technology, "Feeling Fat May Make You Fat, Study Suggests," ScienceDaily, accessed March 20, 2020, *www.sciencedaily.com/releases/2012/08/120808121816.htm*.

16. Ibid.

17. Shelly Grabe, L. Monique Ward, and Janet Shibley Hyde. "The Role of the Media in Body Image Concerns among Women: A Meta-Analysis of Experimental and Correlational Studies." Psychological Bulletin 134, no. 3 (June 2008): 460–76, *https://doi.org/10.1037/0033-2909.134.3.460*.

18. Heather A. Hausenblas and Elizabeth A. Fallon, "Exercise and Body Image: A Meta-Analysis," *Psychology & Health* 21, no. 1 (March 2005): 33–47, *https://doi.org/10.1080/14768320500105270*.

19. Dr. Jake Linardon, "2021 Body Image Statistics: 40 Shocking Body Image Facts," Break Binge Eating, March 6, 2021, *https://breakbingeeating.com/body-image-statistics/*.

20. "Eating Disorder Statistics for Anorexia, Bulimia, Binge Eating," Eating Disorder Hope, February 10, 2021, *https://www.eatingdisorderhope.com/information/statistics-studies*.

21. Andri S. Bjornsson, Elizabeth R. Didie, and Katharine A. Phillips, "Body Dysmorphic Disorder," *Obsessive-Compulsive Spectrum Disorders* 12, no. 2 (June 2010): 221–32, *https://doi.org/10.31887/dcns.2010.12.2/abjornsson*.

22. Talltanic, "10 Craziest Stories of Plastic Surgery Obsessions," YouTube, February 2, 2017, *https://www.youtube.com/watch?v=k-NFfEAyfK4*.

23. Ibid.

24. "Jessica Alves," Wikipedia, Wikimedia Foundation, March 12, 2021, *https://en.wikipedia.org/wiki/Jessica_Alves*.

25. *Diagnostic and Statistical Manual of Mental Disorders: DSM-5* (Arlington, VA: American Psychiatric Association, 2017), 242.

26. Diagnostic and Statistical Manual of Mental Disorders: DSM-5, 243.

27. Letter to Jendayi Harris – Re: Please Approve This Quote from You for The Chubby Church Book 2 in Chapter 26/6 on Body Image, March 22, 2021.

28. John Eldredge and Staci Eldredge, *Captivating: Unveiling the Mystery of a Woman's Soul* (Nashville, TN: Thomas Nelson, 2021), 24.

29. "FastStats – Body Measurements," Centers for Disease Control and Prevention, January 14, 2021, *https://www.cdc.gov/nchs/fastats/body-measurements.htm.*

30. Ibid.

31. "Top 30 Quotes of Martha Beck – Famous Quotes and Sayings: Inspringquotes.us," Inspiring Quotes, accessed March 20, 2021, *https://www.inspiringquotes.us/author/2349-martha-beck.*

32. Anna Carey. "Little Photoshop of Horrors." Independent.ie, (November 30, 2012), *https://www.independent.ie/style/beauty/little-photoshop-of-horrors-26650439.html.*

33. Myles Munroe, *Single, Married, Separated, and Life after Divorce* (Shippensburg, PA: Destiny Image Publishing, 2003), 44.

34. C. B. Taylor, S. Bryson, A. A. Celio Doyle, K. H. Luce, D. Cunning, L. B. Abascal, R. Rockwell, et al, "The Adverse Effect of Negative Comments about Weight and Shape from Family and Siblings on Women at High Risk for Eating Disorders," *Pediatrics* 118, no. 2 (2006): 731–38, *https://doi.org/10.1542/peds.2005-1806.*

35. David Garner, "Body Image in America: Survey Results," Psychology Today, Sussex Publishers, February 1, 1997, *https://www.psychologytoday.com/us/articles/199702/body-image-in-america-survey-results.*

36. Mary Inman, Erica Iceberg, and Laura McKeel, "Do Religious Affirmations, Religious Commitments, or General Commitments Mitigate the Negative Effects of Exposure to Thin Ideals?" *Journal for the Scientific Study of Religion* 53, no. 1 (March 2014): 38–55, *https://doi.org/10.1111/jssr.12089.*

37. "Dana Christmas Story," Campus Firewatch, YouTube video, September 12, 2006, *https://www.youtube.com/watch?v=WzpxaUCOccY.*

38. Dan Barry, "3 Killed in Fire at Seton Hall; Dozens of Students Are Hurt," *The New York Times*, January 20, 2000, *https://www.nytimes. com/2000/01/20/nyregion/3-killed-in-fire-at-seton-hall-dozens-of-students-are-hurt.html.*

39. Bessel van der Kolk, "The Body Keeps the Score: Memory and the Evolving Psychobiology of Posttraumatic Stress," *Harvard Review of Psychiatry*, 1, no. 5 (January 1, 1994): 253-65, *https://pubmed.ncbi.nlm. nih.gov/9384857/.*

40. Ana Sandoiu, "How Can Exercise Improve Body Image?" Medical News Today, MediLexicon International, June 18, 2017, *https://www. medicalnewstoday.com/articles/317958#Post-exercise-positive-effects-can-be-immediate-and-long-lasting.*

41. David Garner, "Body Image in America: Survey Results," Psychology Today, Sussex Publishers, February 1, 1997, *https://www.psychologytoday. com/us/articles/199702/body-image-in-america-survey-results.*

42. Ibid.

43. Rheana Murray, "Where's the Least Body-Positive State in America? You Might Be Surprised," TODAY, May 8, 2018, *https://www.today.com/style/ social-media-affecting-way-we-view-our-bodies-it-s-t128500.*

44. Kay Lazar, "As Women Have Grown Larger, Victoria's Secret Models Have Shrunk," The Boston Globe, January 3, 2020, *https://www. bostonglobe.com/metro/2020/01/02/women-have-grown-larger-victoria-secret-models-have-shrunk/CQKFwaYXg4jbNtAJoWKyBK/story.html.*

45. Carly Cardellino, "16 Surprising Things You Didn't Know about the Victoria's Secret Fashion Show," Cosmopolitan, October 8, 2017, *https://www.cosmopolitan.com/style-beauty/beauty/news/a5045/ things-you-didnt-know-about-the-victorias-secret-fashion-show/.*

46. "Female Promotional Model Averages Infographic," TSM Agency, April 23, 2017, *http://www.blog.tsmagency.com/ average-model-height-and-weight-requirements/.*

Chapter 20: Keys to Whole & Free Health

1. Alina Petre, "Orthorexia: When Healthy Eating Becomes a Disorder," April 2, 2020, *https://www.healthline.com/nutrition/ orthorexia-nervosa-101.*

2. Ibid.

3.   AJ, Chef, and Glen Merzer, The Secrets to Ultimate Weight Loss: a Revolutionary Approach to Conquer Cravings, Overcome Food Addiction, and Lose Weight without Going Hungry (Los Angeles, CA: Hail to the Kale Publishing, 2018), 49.

4.   Douglas and Alan Goldhamer, The Pleasure Trap: Mastering the Hidden Force That Undermines Health & Happiness (Summertown, TN: Healthy Living Publications, 2006),71.

5.   Ibid.

6.   Jamie Locher and Owen Moritz, "Eating While Driving Causes 80% of All Car Accidents, Study Shows," New York Daily News, January 11, 2019, *https://www.nydailynews.com/new-york/ eating-driving-80-car-accidents-study-shows-article-1.427796.*

7.   "Dr. Seuss Quotes and Facts," EasyBib, January 1, 2021, *https://www. easybib.com/guides/quotes-facts-stats/dr-seuss/.*

Invitation to Christ

1.   Douglas Groothuis, *Christian Apologetics: A Comprehensive Case for Biblical Faith* (Downers Grove, IL: IVP Academic, 2011), 503.

2.   Ibid, 500–501.

3.   "Know Jesus," Daystar Television, accessed March 26, 2019. *http://www. daystar.com/prayer/know-jesus/.*

Made in the USA
Monee, IL
30 May 2023

34303121R00214